On Uganda's Terms

A Journal by an American Nurse-Midwife Working for Change in Uganda, East Africa During Idi Amin's Regime

by
Mary M. Hale, RNC, MSN, SRN, SCM

[handwritten: 7-1-13 Peace – Mary M. Hale 2nd edition]

CCB Publishing
British Columbia, Canada

On Uganda's Terms: A Journal by an American Nurse-Midwife Working for Change in Uganda, East Africa During Idi Amin's Regime

Copyright ©2009 by Mary M. Hale
ISBN-13   978-1-926585-13-0
Second Edition

Library and Archives Canada Cataloguing in Publication

Hale, Mary M., 1940-
On Uganda's terms: a journal by an American nurse-midwife working for change in Uganda, East Africa during Idi Amin's regime / written by Mary M. Hale – 2nd ed.
ISBN 978-1-926585-13-0
1. Hale, Mary M., 1940-. 2. Americans--Uganda--Biography.
3. Midwives--Uganda--Biography. 4. Nurses--Uganda--Biography.
5. Maternity nursing--Uganda--Biography.
6. Uganda--Social conditions--1971-1979. I. Title.
RG966.U33H33 2009   362.19'82006761   C2008-908105-6

Publisher: CCB Publishing
             British Columbia, Canada
             www.ccbpublishing.com

This book is dedicated to Colleen Connell, one of the best mothers I know, whose care in putting together this book has been unprecedented. Her computer and editing skills have made this experience a joy for me as the author.

Acknowledgements

We acknowledge the people of Uganda both now and in the past. From their darkness into the light has been a journey of terror, and we share in their hope for the future.

To all of the medical personnel from Mulago Hospital, to Virika Hospital at Fort Portal, to Jinja Hospital and to all of the other hospitals in Uganda, who daily perform "their duty" – thank you and may God bless you always. You are and have been an example to me, one American in the jungle that you took into your hearts.

To Bonnie Kaye, M.Ed., my critic and mentor in my publishing adventure.

To Dr. Kenneth D. Hoellein, M.D., my physician for thirty years ("Just doing my job"), who kept me alive so that I could finish this book.

And lastly, to Dr. John J. Takach, D.D.S., who listened to my countless stories and did not laugh when I told him I was going to be published.

Contents

Preface

It was one month before my escape from Uganda, East Africa thirty years ago. It was the beginning of the Ugandan-Tanzanian war, and the Nilotics started coming from the north of Uganda and the refugees came to our hospital from Rwanda. We were a one hundred and twenty bed hospital in Jinja. As the refugees came, all of the beds were filled with the very ill. The refugees slept on the floors of the wards, pharmacy and lab. The Jinja Hospital nursing pharmacy and lab staff came to the six administrators and asked if they could stay overnight to be there for duty in the morning. We had no food or room and we said "No". But we loaded the Land Rovers with them and set out for the six-mile drive to their village. The staff shouted to turn to the right and they were near their village. We then returned to the hospital.

I stopped at the market and purchased cows' stomachs and intestines for the hospital supper. We washed and rewashed them; but I will never forget the smell of them cooking. The refugees ate them and were satisfied. I ate fruit.

In the morning, the night staff came to me and said that their relief staff had not arrived yet. I had an ominous feeling and we set out to the village to bring them back to the hospital. We traveled down the six miles and turned onto the dirt road where we had left them the night before. There, about 500 feet down the road, the road ran red with blood and off to the right in the elephant grass were their bodies. They had been ambushed by their own Ugandan army and machine-gunned. I ran crying to see if any were alive; but they were all cold.

I remember, after thirty years, what my mind had suppressed, causing me to have nightmares and only three to four hours of sleep per night. I remember it like it was yesterday – the feeling of the sticky blood on my white shoes – the struggle to carry the bodies to the Land Rover for autopsies and burial at the hospital. These were people that I had loved and worked with for the last ten years – all gone. Some of the "eighteen" were pregnant.

This book is meant as a tribute to their lives. They were simple Ugandans serving their fellow men at a Ugandan hospital under the Ministry of Health thirty years ago.

I reread this book and often think of their "daily duty" and their sacrifice.

Introduction

Why now? Why would I want to write my story now – 30 years after it happened? Because Idi Amin is dead now – he passed away in 2003. President for life Field Marshal Al Hadj Dr. Idi Amin Dada, VC, DSO, Lord of all the Beasts of the earth and fishes of the sea, King of Scots, and Conqueror of the British Empire in Africa in general and Uganda in particular signed my work permit that began my years of medical service for the Ugandan Ministry of Health. I fulfilled my promise of 30 years ago – I would not write my book until he died. Well, "Bon Voyage Idi!"

I retired from Albert Einstein Healthcare Network in Philadelphia, Pennsylvania on June 3, 2006 after 27 years of being a nurse in Pediatrics and Obstetrics. As you probably know, nurses are always very busy people. Nursing is integrated into my being, so most of this book will be about what happened in the hospital and medical communities in northwestern and southern Uganda during the years 1964 through 1969 and 1974 through 1979.

Uganda is located in Eastern Africa. It is bordered to the north by the Sudan, to the east by Kenya, Tanzania to the south, Rwanda and Burundi to the southwest and the Democratic Republic of the Congo to the west.

After my retirement on June 3, 2006, I had to recuperate for four months in order to start remembering the memoirs for this book. Helen and Paul Wagabaza of Madison, Wisconsin have been a great help to me in remembering.

The Reason

I didn't know if I wanted to remember. I had seen it all – public executions, the beatings and shootings, death and destruction that I didn't think were possible. I had looked into the face of evil – Idi Amin as he signed my ex-patriate contract, upon my return from nursing and midwifery training, to improve the health and well being of mothers and children. We started the first Postgraduate Pediatric Program in Uganda, East Africa. I remember overhearing the Senior Nursing Officer, Lucy Walusimbi, telling Idi Amin "I need this woman".

Mr. Henry Kyemba, Minister of Health, went into Amin's office first to speak privately to the President. I sat outside the office and could hear every word between Amin and Mr. Kyemba, as the Minister tried to convince Amin that I was needed by the Ministry of Health to start the first Postgraduate Pediatric Course while their tutor was still in England finishing her nursing tutorial course. Their meeting went on for four hours.

Amin's first concern was that I would write a book about him based on incorrect information and increase the prejudice Americans held against him. I promised him that I would not write anything about him until after his death. And so I kept my promise – it's been thirty years, and Amin died in August, 2003. At that time, I was asking for a work permit. I had been back in Uganda since my nursing and midwifery training under a visitor's visa; but working with the Ugandan women and children.

Amin signed the work permit and wished me "Good Luck" as he shook my hand.

I write this sitting in my home, filled with African art and memories of a time that filled me with terror and longing to come home again. But, I could not turn my back on the need of the Ugandan people. I remember as if it were yesterday.

Could I as a white nurse midwife make a difference alone in black Uganda?

I am the only child of Irish Catholic parents who were in their late forties when I was born. Of my early life, I can only say that in my late teens I had to sever the apron strings and do something to fulfill my goal of helping people through public service, all the while enhancing health, well being and the quality of life. My work in Uganda thirty years ago aimed to fulfill these goals. My motivation for going to Uganda was based on medical facts that in Africa a child dies of malaria every thirty seconds (two million children every year). Yearly maternal and neonatal Tetanus (MNT) claimed the lives of almost 180,000 infants and 30,000 mothers (TIME Magazine). How would I find the power we all have to save a life? I always remember the saying from the Talmud "If you can save one life, you can save a generation."

In doing my research for the possibility of working in developing countries, I contacted the Ugandan Embassy in Washington, DC. They sent me some information regarding the Ugandan culture and the health and welfare of the people. Upon receiving this information I decided that it was time to take action.

My first five years under Dr. Milton Obote (1964-1969) were very peaceful despite the death and disease of ignorance, as I worked as an accountant to try and get a mission hospital out of debt. I learned the language and customs and learned to love the Ugandan people. I found out that although we are diverse, it is important to realize that humans everywhere share certain features of life in common.

After I spent a few years at Holy Family Hospital (Virika) at Fort Portal, I met for the second time a very influential person by the name of Lucy Walusimbi, who was Uganda's Senior Nursing Officer. She was in charge of all the Ugandan registered nurses and midwives. She gave her heart and soul as their leader. She stated that I was a "people person" and not a "book person". She encouraged me to return to the U.S. and study nursing and midwifery. She said that nursing in Uganda without midwifery does not meet the needs of the Ugandan woman.

I returned to the U.S. and took nursing at Philadelphia General Hospital, staffed the Detention Ward for 6 months and then went to England to study midwifery. I chose England because their midwifery program was only 18 months in duration compared to a four-year program in the United States at that time. Then I returned to Uganda to teach their first Postgraduate Pediatric Program and nursing leadership skills to give these young Ugandan women a responsibility in caring for their children. It was at this time that Idi Amin rose to power. When I was in Jinja doing what I was contracted to do, rumors did abound and gunfire was heard at night during

Idi Amin's regime in Uganda (1975-1979). Amin's time in power can be summed up in his own words "There is no incense for something rotting."

It helps to understand some history as to how Uganda evolved to Amin. So how did the Colonial Government emerge in this East African country? According to Giles Foden's book "The Last King of Scotland", Arab slave traders appeared early in the 18th century. "Uganda's Colonial period began with the arrival of John Hanning Speke in 1862. After Speke, a large number of European explorers, evangelical missionaries, and a number of merchants (the Imperial British East African Company) migrated to Uganda. Around the period of 1885-1887, newly converted Christians in Uganda were being killed by burning, castration and dismemberment. Fights flared between the Christians and the supporters of the Kabaka (King of Buganda, one of the many Ugandan provinces). The Catholics favored French or German colonialism while the Anglicans favored the British.

Uganda continued as a Protectorate of the British rule until independence in 1962. In 1903, Joseph Chamberlain, the British Secretary for the Colonies, offered the country to Theodore Herzl and the World Zionist Organization as a possible Jewish State. They refused the offer of residence; the Zionists were alarmed by the interest from Palestine."

In a study of the religious history of Uganda, I was surprised by a story (available only through oral tradition) of the Ugandan martyrs of the late 1800's. There were 22 young men who served as pages in the court of King Mutesa of one of the Ugandan provinces. The King approached the young men for sexual favors. All 22 were of different religious backgrounds but strong in their faith.

They were beaten and chained and marched 20 miles to where they were burned at the stake. Pope Pius XII was so impressed by their story that he canonized all 22 young men, despite their different religious backgrounds. The deep religious spirit of the Ugandan martyrs remained with me throughout my period of service to their country.

Could I, as an individual, make a difference on Uganda's terms?

The Location

According to an Information Sheet released from the Ugandan Embassy in the U.S., Uganda is about the size of the state of Oregon and is situated in East Africa. It lies astride the equator on the central African plateau nearly 900 miles from the east coast. This landlocked country is bordered on the west by the Democratic Republic of the Congo, the north by the Sudan, the east by Kenya, and the south by Tanzania and Rwanda.

The county is diagonally bisected by the River Nile and the lakes and waterways of the Lake Kioga system. Lake Victoria, which forms some of the southern border, is the second largest inland lake in the world and the source of the Nile River.

Uganda is a country of magnificent scenery and was described by early travelers as the "Pearl of Africa's Crown". It consists of the rolling savannah green plains in the northern plateau, the Bufumbira volcanoes in the extreme southwest, the snow peaks of the Rwenzori Mountains, Mount Elgon in the east, an extinct volcano, the forest in the southwest and southeast whose trees soar to a lofty 150 feet, the hot springs of the southwest, the Sipi and Kabalaga Falls in the east and north respectively.

Despite its tropical location, Uganda's climate is tempered by an average altitude of 3,000 to 6,000 feet. Much of the country enjoys an average annual temperature of 71 degrees Fahrenheit and a good prospect of obtaining about 50 inches of rainfall every year. The country's climate is often described as a European summer all year round.

With such a generally agreeable climate, it is not surprising that the first impression of a visitor to Uganda is one of greenness and the reddish-orange soil. Lake Victoria has a marked effect on the climate of southern Uganda and a belt of generous rainfall along the north shore of the lake. This supports the neighboring tropical rainforest. Tall elephant grass grows on the land and even at the driest time of the year, the countryside retains its green freshness.

Substantial mineral deposits of cobalt, copper, and limestone are among Uganda's natural resources. Its location at the source of the Nile makes it a potentially potent source of hydroelectric power.

Agriculture accounts for virtually all of Uganda's export earnings. Coffee and cotton are its major export crops, with coffee providing more than 90 percent of export earnings. Other agricultural products include tea, bananas, sugar cane, corn and cassava.

Most industry in Uganda is related to agriculture, such as cotton ginning, coffee, curing and manufacture of agricultural tools. The industrial sector also produces building and construction materials including cement, angle bars, corrugated iron sheets, and paint.

When I arrived in Uganda, it had about 20,000 miles of roads, one fifth of which are paved. Most radiate from Kampala, the capital and largest city. It also has about

800 miles of railroad and an international airport in Entebbe on the shore of Lake Victoria.

Uganda is a republic headed by a President with executive powers. The President appoints Cabinet Ministers. The National Resistance Council is the supreme authority of government. The Ugandan Judiciary operates as an independent branch of government. An independent Public Service Commission appoints all officers and defense forces that have their own commissions.

H. E. Yoweri Museveni is President and Minister of Defense. The honorable Dr. Samson Kiseka is the Prime Minister at this time.

The early history of Uganda is characterized by the interaction and intermixture of diverse groups of immigrants from elsewhere in Africa and these migrations involved linguistic groups of Bantu language speakers from southwest and southeast, Nilotes moving southward along the Nile Valley, Sudanic language speakers from the Northwest, and the Hermitic groups from the southern highlands of Ethiopia moving southwest-wards.

By the nineteenth century, most of the Uganda communities comprised different mixtures of immigrant communities and combined in different ways the traditions, experiences, and the inventions of the component groups. Around Lake Victoria agricultural communities tended to form themselves into kingdom states. In the west, pastoral people often established aristocratic states, which included agricultural people. In the north, people adopted small scale and flexible institutions for their own government. Late in the nineteenth century European travelers were often impressed and surprised by the complexity of the kingdom governments, which resembled similar institutions in Europe. On the other hand, they found it difficult to deal with even more complex segmented communities.

During the course of the "scramble for Africa" in the late nineteenth century, a British Protectorate was established in 1893 over the Kingdom of Buganda. By 1914 the Protectorate, whose name was now rendered Uganda, had spread to present boundaries of the country.

Uganda became independent in 1962. From 1962 to 1966, a dual system of unitary and federal government was practiced with Mutesa II, King of Buganda as President, and Milton Obote as Prime Minister. In 1966, the Prime Minister deposed Mutesa II and the former became Executive President. The following year Uganda became a republic and all kingdoms were abolished.

In 1971, Idi Amin took over power, after leading a military coup and ruled the country up to 1979. Ugandans witnessed a brutal and murderous reign of terror. The brutality of the government and its army resulted in widespread insecurity and murder of thousands of Ugandans. In 1979, exiled guerilla groups backed by Tanzanian troops ousted Idi Amin. Exiled groups founded the Ugandan National Liberation Front (UNLF), which formed a brief interim government in which Yusuf Lule and Godfrey Binaisa served as President respectively.

The National Resistance Movement Government follows an economic strategy of mixed economy, whereby; private entrepreneurs carry out the majority of economic activities. The state takes part in selected fulcrum-like sectors that it can use to guide the economy as a whole toward the desired goals. The aim of the government is to build an independent, integrated, and self sustaining national economy whereby the economy is oriented to produce, as much as possible, those commodities, goods, or equipment that will enable productive sectors, especially industry and agriculture to support each other.

The government encourages investments by investors abroad. A law exists to protect such investment as well as give incentives to those who wish to invest in Uganda. The Foreign Investment Protection Act of 1964 and the subsequent Decree of 1977, give details of what the investors need to do before they start their projects in Uganda. The law provides for a committee of senior officers who are supposed to examine the nature of the proposed investment and determine whether it is in line with the country's development objectives. If the committee is satisfied, it makes recommendations to the Minister of Finance who signs a Certificate of Approved status, thus allowing the investors the right to remit dividends and interest on any money they might have borrowed from abroad to finance the project in the country.

It should be emphasized, however, that each project has to be discussed with the government on a case-by-case basis to insure that its future operations are in line with government's economic objectives and will produce those goods or services the country considers a priority.

On Uganda's Terms

The Culture

Looking at "Cultural Anthropology" by Barbara D. Miller, some say culture is attitude. I say culture embraces all that we are, where we were, and where we are going. It involves kinship and language.

When I first landed at Entebbe airport in the sixties, I realized I was far from home – no white faces at all and the soil was reddish orange. The African children, who greeted me, started rubbing my arms to see if I was black underneath like them. I said, "No, God didn't love me as much as He loved you. He left you in the oven longer." They were delighted at my response.

As I learned the Rutooro dialect at the local catecumenate with the young children, I learned that their proverbs were the best way to get a clue as to their teachings. "Kamu, kamu, nigwo muganda." which means "One by one makes a bundle." We have the saying "A stitch in time saves nine" in America. In time of war, "Akanyoni, ka hara, kasoma nukwu obwire." which translates as "The little bird from afar, as he pecks at the seeds, watches the sun."

The first proverb that I took to my heart was "Okuha nomuha, nizo ngonzi itafwa." which means "When one gives love to another, love never dies."

Just to give you an idea of the simplicity and goodness of the Ugandan people, I recall the following account.

When I first went to Jinja Hospital, the news was circulated that I was not married at that time. The suitors lined up by the hundreds over the next month. I was wined and dined in the local hotels and I knew the ultimate reason – the green immigration card to get to America-by all means!

One of the "love letters" was started by the phrase "Dear Lovely" which would become my clown's name many years later, as I became the Delaware Valley's first Public Health Teaching Clown in Philadelphia.

The staff would always greet me in the morning when I came on duty – "Oraire Ota" which means, "How are you?" I would answer, "Ndoho kurungi" which means, "All is well." Even though the night might have been peppered with gunfire, they were always polite.

Weddings were always a huge event. The very wealthy couples always had a European or American-like wedding. The people with limited income always had numerous events that were worth remembering. I remember one of our staff midwives with limited income was worried right up to the day of the event what the main course would be – beef, pork, warthog or fish. It could be anything, even vegetables. What a blessing – a huge Nile perch washed up on the shores of Lake Victoria deceased of natural causes; but freshly deceased. It was stuffed with vegetables and cooked for hours in hot coals underground. Everyone ate well and no one got ill. We enjoyed banana beer. Bananas are placed in a hollowed-out wooden boat and left to ferment. The beer is very gritty and a lot like our porridge (corn or maize flour) or cereal. Wedding gifts are often money for the young couple. Relatives and friends come from near and far for the three to four day celebration.

When the Ugandan doctors had returned from Russia after their medical training, they usually had a Russian woman accompanying them as their wife. The Russian nurses were only trained in one specialty such as Pediatrics. This always made it difficult for the supervisors trying to staff the hospital with supervisors during the evening and night shifts. The specialties of Obstetrics, Medical-Surgical, or Psychiatry were usually uncovered. The staffing problem always put a lot of responsibility on the staff nurses working in those particular areas.

As we would pass the doctors' houses, we could hear the family fights about cultural misunderstandings. Usually everything was communicated in Russian even though the national language was English. Sometimes the Russian nurses would have to attend banquets honoring Amin and various administrative personnel. They would be exposed to fillets of Nile perch and gumbo soup made from okra and crayfish. The biggest surprise for them was the dudu platter – bee larvae, large green bush crickets, grasshoppers, cicadas, and flying ants, all fried with a little oil and salt.

Uganda reminded me of the constant changing of the color of the chameleon. The flowers were frangipani, Bird of Paradise, elephant grass, pagoda flower, prickly pear, poinsettia, cacti, and shrimp plants galore. The national bird – the Crested Crane – has a yellow crest, a black and white face, long beak, and eyes that looked in complete surprise.

The national costume of Uganda was very varied in design for the women. Basically, the Basuti was a Victorian style long dress with puffy sleeves and a cumberbun. Many of the Basutis were of African prints. The men wore a simple white long gown with a suit jacket.

I remember when I first arrived in Uganda and we were traveling up to Fort Portal – 200 miles from Kampala, the Land Rover was full of men and women in their national costumes. As we curved around a dirt road in the Land Rover, we came across a circle of baboons in the middle of the road. They looked as though they were having a conference. All I could remember was the circle of their red bottoms. The driver stopped the Land Rover and waited for the baboons to move into the bush. I always remember the reverence that the Ugandans had for the animals. Queen Elizabeth National Park was full of elephants, giraffe, lions, gazelles, warthogs, buffalo, monkeys and snakes. During Amin's regime, especially during the Ugandan-Tanzanian War the animals gradually disappeared, as the soldiers ate them.

Most of the animals in the park, as well as the farm animals, had to scrounge for their own food. We would see cattle grazing on sticks of grass and the chickens looked as if they were eating stones. Meat, therefore, was very tough. I had brought a pressure cooker with me and still found it tough to chew.

One time when I went home for furlough, I was on Ethiopian Airlines. This was during the time of Haile Selassie, Emperor of Ethiopia. The planes were very richly decorated with gold brocades on the walls. The meals were magnificent. The stewardesses were dressed in gorgeous silk saris and were very gracious. One of the stewardesses placed a meal in front of me and I thought I was in heaven. I started to cut the meat as I had been conditioned to do after five years of nothing but "the tough stuff". I cut into the meat with such strength that it flew onto the airplane's floor. The stewardess immediately saw what had happened and brought me a new platter. She took the other plate and asked if I could reach for the other steak on the floor, so she could take it away. I told her that I had already eaten it, as I was so hungry.

The jacket of Elizabeth Bagaaya Nyabongo's book describes her as "the embodiment of Ugandan culture, a three-time exile and active resistance leader. She reflected the evolution of African politics from the rule of ancient monarchies to the turbulence of Ugandan independence in 1963. She was born into a royal family in a country province called Toro. She was the daughter of King George Matthew Kamurasi Rickiiki III. She came of age in the midst of pageantry and privilege, a princess of Toro. From her early days in a Toro primary school, she was even taught the primitive art of cleaning elephant grass and digging with a simple hoe to plant banana trees. She went to a top boarding school, where she prepared for her powerful and time-honored role as the "Batebe" or Princess Royal. She was one of the first African women to graduate from Cambridge University. She became the first woman lawyer in Uganda. Her father lived to see her triumph, but he died shortly thereafter unleashing a powerful struggle that changed the course of East African history." When Elizabeth's father was laid out for viewing, thousands of Ugandans passed by the bier in homage. He was wrapped in bark cloth, except for his face. Bark cloth comes from a special tree called omuoma where a small piece of bark is pounded and watered until it grows into a strong cloth-like fabric.

Wealth in Uganda is measured not by your purse but by the people in your life – your relatives. When an African dies, his wealth can be measured by the manner in which he is mourned. The Omukama, or King of Toro, was mourned for nine days.

When Elizabeth's brother, Patrick, was crowned the new King of Toro, dictator Milton Obote's coup de-etat launched an era of unprecedented terror.

Elizabeth was offered a modeling assignment in England and appeared on the covers of many magazines such as Vogue. She later had a film career. You had to see Elizabeth to appreciate her beauty. She was over 6 feet tall and weighed about 120 pounds. Her hair was styled in that of the day but when her father died, her head was shaved in sorrow. She had light brown skin with an oval face and almond-shaped eyes.

When General Idi Amin overthrew Dr. Obote, he asked Elizabeth to return to Uganda as Ambassador at Large and Minister of Foreign Affairs. She returned for a career in public service. Elizabeth had many diplomatic successes including a time at the United Nations. Amin turned against her and forced her to flee to Kenya. She returned only after Amin's fall. Both she and her husband, a commercial pilot, fought for the liberation of Uganda through the National Resistance Movement. President Museveni, after overthrowing Amin, appointed her Amabassor to the United Nations. From the Mountains of the Moon to a life of international diplomacy, she truly provides invaluable perspective on the mind of modern Africa. She is truly one of the reasons Uganda is still called "The Pearl of Africa's Crown".

Elizabeth's Empaako was Akiiki. Empaako is the Kitoro word for an endearing name such as a pet name. This word is not a nickname. All the Batoro people have Empaakos (pet names). Some names are only for men or women; others are for both. Some of the names are as follows: Akiiki, Amoti, Abwoli, Atenyi, Adyeri, and Apoli. It was a real honor for me to have been given an Empaako, Akiiki (the kind one). Empaako's are hardly ever given to white people.

As referred to in Giles Foden's book, "The Last King of Scotland", some of the names of the villages are from oral tradition, such as the village of Namusagali. The village was named, since the people were amazed at the train when it first arrived. They would go to see the train and greet it by saying "Namusa Gali" which means, "I am greeting the long bicycle with smoke". They named their village after that greeting.

When the white people came, the villagers thought they wanted to steal their fish from the river. So they called the river "Semuliki", that is "river without fish".

To the people of Uganda, dancing comes naturally to both young and old. Indeed it is a means of which culture and history have been passed from one generation to another.

The country's impressive cultural heritage is abundantly demonstrated by the success of Uganda's famed "Heartbeat of Africa" dancing troop, which have won worldwide acclaim on its frequent tours abroad, so much so that traditional dancing is considered a great attraction and entertainment for visitors.

Language and kinship tell it all.

On Uganda's Terms

The Money

In 1964, I went to Uganda as a secretary and accountant for a private missionary hospital serving outpatients and inpatients in the western part of Uganda in a small town called Fort Portal (Kabarole). A very old Catholic cathedral stood in the center of town. Two hospitals – one Protestant, Kabarole Hospital, stood looking at the Mountains of the Moon. The Catholic hospital, Virika, stood opposite the old cathedral. Both served the Batoro people as well as they could. The following story illustrates this fact.

Yosufu had been born in the village and brought into our hospital at Virika very ill. The infant was also very premature and had tetanus. Local midwives do the village deliveries. When they cut the cord, custom dictates that they cover the cord with cow dung. The bacteria caused the tetanus with its progressive and often fatal seizures and sequale. Due to the expense of the tetanus immune globulin, the hospital administrators had to request that the medicine be sent from London, England via express. In 1966 it cost $90 – and almost always it arrived too late. In Yosufu's case, it did arrive too late to the sorrow of both parents.

My job was in the admission and discharge office, along with Anthony, who was my assistant and translator.

It was my job to try and get payment for the hospitalization from the family. I had learned Swahili prior to entering Uganda and utilized this in my dealings with the public. Five years later, one of my loyal students told me that I should not be speaking Swahili, as it was fishmongers and prostitutes language. I took this to heart and attended the local daily Mugigi (catecuminate), where Fr. Archangelo taught Rutooro, the local dialect, and religion. Uganda's population, like that of most African countries, is distributed among so many tribal and subregional populations that there is no majority group, just larger and smaller minorities.

Now money, as we all know, is the root of all evil. But it certainly helps to have it as is emphasized by the following. In 1964, when I first went to Uganda, we had a layover in West Germany. For some reason we had to be body searched when reembarking to our final destination in Uganda, East Africa. I was led into a dressing room by a female customs officer, where she stayed with me until I started to undress. I was down to my underwear, when there was a commotion in the next cubicle. She simply stated, "Get dressed" and my close call was over. Apparently there had been a drug bust in the next cubicle. I knew that I was probably going to have to ride my way out of a few close calls, so I had stashed $600 in varied bills in my girdle. This type of close call came when I had to purchase an airline ticket out of Nairobi, Kenya for my escape in 1979. My good friend, Helen Wagabaza, had started with the paralysis of her hands. She had given whatever meat was available to her six children. The lack of vitamin B12 from the meat caused her to come down with a peripheral neuropathy. She had to travel to Kenya to get the vitamin B12 injections and she smuggled my $600 over the Kenyan border to purchase an open ticket from Nairobi to London for me when the time was right for my escape.

Thirty years ago the East African shilling was equivalent to 7 shillings to the American dollar.

When I worked at Jinja Hospital, the diet of the patients was always in question. The pediatric patients always needed dry milk to get their porridge (corn or maize flour) down. Many of the children had diseases like kwashiokor and marasmus – protein calorie malnutrition and starvation. Their big bellies on stick-like legs are the result of parasite infestation.

After a few years of trying to beg, borrow or steal the dry milk, I waited until my furlough and I stopped at the Save the Children organization in London. We arranged for the donation of 5 tons of dried skim milk, which I witnessed being unloaded from the plane in Entebbe airport in Uganda. The Ugandan army unloaded the milk and some of the paper bags fell and exposed the dried milk onto the airfield tarmac and the wind just blew it away. Some of the supply was carted off to the army barracks for their coffee and porridge. The children did get a small amount.

I had to wait until my next furlough to discuss this theft with the Save the Children organization in London. Nothing could be spoken or written while in Uganda for obvious reasons. When I arrived in London I had thought of a way to disguise the dried skim milk as medicine to get it past the army. We decided to color the dried skim milk with Gentian Violet – a dye used on the umbilical cord after birth. When the shipment landed, they did steal some of the bags as usual and when they opened them they realized they could not use them without detection.

The children received their milk and were able to eat their porridge.

Another time that money was involved was the 10 million dollars of U.S. aid that our country was giving at the time of the 1960's and 1970's. Most of the money was used to buy arms and filtered into the Ugandan army. Beer and spirits were free flowing with both the higher and lower ranks of the army. It even filtered to the men at the roadside who sat there drunk, while some of their wives who had just had a C-section two days previously were now tilling the fields with the newborn on their backs.

The village economics was the basis of survival. I can only write about my nursing staff and how they survived. The staff, which worked at Jinja Hospital, earned a monthly salary, which was enough to buy a pair of shoes via Magendo – the black market. Most of the staff had shambas in the village, which would be 30-60 miles away from the hospital where they lived. They would go to the village on their days off and bring back their matooke (green bananas), soyabeans, veggies, which they grew, and sometimes they brought back meat.

On all of our Land Rover travels, we would take very little money due to the robberies. The 200-mile route from Kampala to Fort Portal, where Virika Hospital was located, was a danger both physically and mentally. The road was dirt and had many twists and turns as it headed to the Mountains of the Moon (Rwenzori Mountains), which are snow-covered. It was often said at the hospital that many miscarriages came to women who traveled that road in a Land Rover. When you were stopped along the road by any of the local bandits, you never knew if you would have a Land Rover left, but you were always separated from your cash.

They never kidnapped anyone in those early days. We also had to be careful of what we ate along the route. Some of the huts that served food were notorious for food poisoning. If we stopped at a local stand, it was always to buy boiled eggs, tea and a banana in the skin. I remember in 1976 coming back from one of my furloughs in America, I drank the water at Entebbe airport. Two days later after bouts of diarrhea, I collapsed and was admitted to the "Grade A" pavilion at the Jinja Hospital. After being rehydrated, I awoke to see one of the nurses polishing a metal, luer-lock needle on a pumice stone. Apparently my IV had infiltrated and she was preparing another infusion. When she saw my frightened look, she stated that the needle was going to be boiled before being inserted into my vein. I thought it over and then asked what IV fluids were being infused. She stated, "Ringers Lactate" and I asked her to give me the bottle of IV fluids and a cup. I proceeded to drink it and another liter as well. I cured myself.

As I recuperated, I got to know all about the private pavilion into which I had been admitted. I noticed that when one of the African doctors would come to do rounds, all of the African nurses would disappear and only the Asian and Russian nurses were left to assist him. I remembered this and filed it away in my brain.

Later, after I moved into the nurses' hostel in Jinja Hospital, I would look out of my window through the lattice brickwork into the "Grade A" pavilion and had a clear view of the nurses' station, as well as the surrounding private rooms. Early in the morning the African doctor would come for his morning rounds and help himself to the narcotics. All the African nurses were petrified of him and would run and hide. I would see this occur every day until I had the locks changed on the medicine cabinets and confronted him. He told me the medical staff had to work under extenuating circumstances. During Idi Amin's regime, doctors had not been paid in 13 months and they were using their tabs at The Crested Crane Hotel. Most of them were alcoholics and on some form of drugs to decrease the stress, isolation, and threat of having to treat Idi Amin during one of his spontaneous visits to the area. When I read Giles Foden's book, "The Last King of Scotland," I couldn't help imagine what these doctors were going through with all of the loose ends and insidious betrayals they were living.

After I encouraged him to go to drug counseling (whatever that meant at the time), we became the best of friends. When I went to Entebbe airport for a furlough to America for 3 months, he accompanied me to the airport. He gave me a letter to read on the plane. He really felt that I was not going to return. His letter stated that we only have two emotions really, love and fear, with a circle of balance surrounding both of them. His balance he stated was off on the fear factor, and he was very afraid of the political situation in Uganda.

We would hear the tropical birds singing in the morning and gunfire at night. When I first landed at Entebbe, I stayed at a local convent that had a hostel. It had an inner courtyard with tropical flowers and birds. I thought it was out of this world. The hospital had a Land Rover and transported me with no financial worries to Fort Portal in Northwestern Uganda, located some 100 miles from the Democratic Republic of the Congo, as the crow flies. Later during my tour of duty, I would travel the route once a month and stay at the same hostel. During Amin's regime, there was a fuel shortage – most of the fuel was diverted to the army. My trips were to check out the antibiotic situation for our hospital. At one time, there was only one antibiotic, Gentamycin, in the whole country.

I would get my breakfast early and pick up my bagged lunch and travel by taxi to Kampala, some 18 miles of Tarmac, to pick up the bus at the bus park for Fort Portal. Sometimes I would get there and find out that there was no petrol. I would travel back to the hostel only to try again the next morning. It all depended on supply and demand and money.

At times, I would take a taxi if nothing else were available. The taxi ride was something else. Each taxi was about the size of our sedan. The usual number of passengers was 10 and above. My heart was in my mouth every time we took a curve around the mountain roads. Usually half way during the journey one of the passengers would often say "Ningonza Kusessa" (I have to pass water). The taxi would stop and everyone would get out letting the person out. Trips at that time were about 50 Uganda shillings ($7 American dollars) for a 200-mile trip to the Rwenzori Mountains (Mountains of the Moon). The mountains were snow covered and on the equator, but the height was 6,000 feet. My trips to Entebbe in search of medications were not in vain. I often heard in Entebbe and around the hospital in Fort Portal that it must be necessary, as the "Muzungu" (the white one) traveled the 200 miles in the Land Rover to request the necessary drugs.

We were always short of supplies. One time we had an obstetric patient who hemorrhaged with no chance of a blood transfusion or blood expander. I ran to the lab, knowing her blood type, and stole 2 pints of O positive blood that had been donated by the family member of a man who was going to have an amputation in the morning. The woman survived after receiving the 2 pints of blood. In the morning I went to see the man whose blood I had appropriated. The Ugandan people are basically a good people who have been misguided politically over a long period of years.

They would die rather than offend an expatriate. This is probably due to the internal repercussions. The gentleman listened while I told him about his blood and simply said, "Well, I guess we have to get more of my relatives to donate for my surgery." No request for payment for the blood was ever brought up. The respect for the decisions that were made by the expatriate staff was always quite evident.

When I first arrived in Jinja, I was supposed to be given a house. Since I came by myself and did not want a whole house, the Ugandan government placed me in the Crested Crane Hotel. I had a single room on the first floor just opposite the telephone exchange. Most of the hotel guests were upper level army officers. Being in a strange place, I listened very carefully to what I could overhear without being observed. The room above mine had two army officers who spoke fluent Swahili. One night after dark, they had their windows open and were discussing what it would be like to rape the Muzungu (the white one). I locked my door, and placed a chair under my doorknob. I began to pack and stayed awake all night. There was no one scheduled to staff the telephone exchange all night. I thought what psychological warfare – the telephones in the staff room rang all night. I called the Senior Nursing Officer in the morning and arranged to move into the Nurses' Hostel, housing staff midwives at the time. As I was moving my luggage out of the hotel, the two army officers were standing on the hotel steps. The one said to the other "Now, see what you have done." I called the Minister of Health, the Minister of Education and the Minister of Internal Affairs and told them the latest story. I found out later that the army officers were stripped of their rank and subjected to the army barracks as privates.

I was relieved to live in the Nurses' Hostel at no charge, as I felt guilty signing the invoices for the 3,000 Uganda shillings per month at the Crested Crane Hotel for room and board. I could not justify living on that scale, when I was there to treat poor mothers and children.

There were incidences at the Nurses' Hostel, since my students for the Postgraduate Pediatric Course had not yet arrived to live and study in that Nurses' Hostel. I had a room with a common bathroom, shared with the other staff nurses living there at the time. The male doctors and other men would come and go all night. The light bulbs in the hallway were stolen due to the lack of everything. In the middle of the night, I went across the hall to the bathroom and ran into the arms of a male about 6'6" much to my fright.

The staff nurses were trying to get rid of me, since when my students came, they would have to move out. So, I was their enemy. They tried in many ways to "remove" me from their village. I used to collect my food from the "Grade A" pavilion kitchen, since they cooked for the European patients. One noon, I had a woman with a very difficult delivery and I lost my appetite. I went to the kitchen to collect my food and found it all dried out. I took it over to the Nurses' Hostel, fed it to the dog, and later that day the dog died.

Here is another example of their attempts. I would often wear white rubber boots during deliveries. I had cleaned them and left them in a safe place at the hospital. One day I tried to put them on and had difficulty. I pulled my foot out and there was a snake in the boot. Thank God I wasn't bitten.

Money was always a pressing problem when Amin cut the salaries of all of the expatriates. The White Fathers would give me a rabbit and vegetables once in awhile; otherwise I ate what my Ugandan students ate. My salary was a gallon of unpasteurized milk, and a dozen of small pullet eggs along with the monetary remuneration. I would go to Kampala once a month to stand in line to collect my supplies of a kilo of sugar, a bar of soap, and a bottle of cooking oil. When I returned to Jinja, I would share the sugar and the bar of soap with the students and the hospital. For example, the bar of soap was 1-1/2 feet long and 4 inches wide. We would cut small pieces and divide it for the hand washing in the wards. When Amin had donated a dental clinic about a mile from the main hospital for use as a Children's Ward, we saw a big change in infection rates. The children were treated in the Adult Wards with no facility for isolation at all. When we opened the two building pediatric ward, one building was for isolation for typhoid fever, meningitis, TB, smallpox, and other communicable diseases. The other building was for the Pediatric Clinic and all non-infectious diseases. The building had one toilet, which was usually broken with leaves and sticks.

I approached the Jinja Lions Club and got donations of cement, bricks, and labor to build six connected pit latrines with shower facilities and a cement shelf for diaper changes. One of the children, an orphan, Stella Maris, was raised in the hospital. She was immunized, bathed, fed, nurtured and slept within the hospital until we saved enough of our salaries to send her to boarding school. Stella Maris was originally found in the gutter of downtown Jinja breastfeeding on her deceased mother.

Since only 1/3 of my salary was allowed outside of the country, when I left Uganda, I made a promise to pay the school fees for Stella Maris' education. In those days, in Uganda the family paid for grades one through twelve (primary to secondary school). Technical training schools, colleges, and universities were paid for by the government with subsidies. Now she is a Pediatrician. She works at the same hospital that she was raised in.

Most of the children's food was grown at the hospital's "Mwanamugimu" ("You have fallen into good things") garden. We planted passion fruits, sweet potatoes, peanuts, greens, corn and bananas just to name a few. The garden came first followed by the building of the pit latrines, which were placed a public health safe distance away from the garden.

I remember a funny incident when they were building. They forgot to cover the deep holes when building the latrines, and as I was teaching in the garden a barking dog fell into the hole, which was about 20 feet deep. We called the local fire department and they arrived with a bucket, a rope and a net. They proceeded to lower the bucket. The grateful dog climbed into the bucket immediately and they hoisted him up to the surface and he got out of there very fast. He had his tail between his legs and was yelping.

When I returned to America in 1979, I was deposed in Washington, DC. For 3 days I stayed in a local hotel with a typewriter and wrote of all the horrors and abuses I had seen. Years later one of the interns that I had worked with at Jinja Hospital visited me in Philadelphia to request that I go with him to Washington, DC to try and get the aid reinstated. We traveled to Washington and went to numerous departments. The aid was reinstated and now that doctor is a Member of Parliament in Uganda. Doctor stated that they were on a very tight budget and any amount would help out greatly. He assured me that the money would go toward health and welfare as well as education.

The Politics

I have seen peace and I have seen pain. Just like in Giles Foden's book, from the foothills of the Mountains of the Moon, we heard the bagpipes. Scottish paraphernalia, kilts, sporrans, white and red checkered gaiters, drums and pipes came over the hill marching along the dirt road, just as if it were the most normal thing in the world. They were the border patrol complete with bright cummerbunds and on each head sat a tall red fez with a black tassel.

How did we come to this? How did Amin who is responsible for over 300,000 deaths come to power? The most accurate account of the Ugandan terror comes from "The Drum" (the National Newspaper of Kenya). Amin himself states, "All men are both good and bad and presidents are also men. We must respect our presidents even if they become so bad that we have to remove them. We made them presidents, if they are bad, we only have ourselves to blame." The words are those of Idi Amin, dictator of the landlocked Uganda for nine years.

Idi Amin Dada was born on January 1, 1924 of a peasant family at Arua, in Uganda's remote West Nile District belonging to the small dominantly Muslim Kakwa tribe. In his late teens, he joined the British-Officered Kings African Rifles where his splendid physique made him an ideal recruit for the tough, highly disciplined corps, which fought with distinction in the Second World War.

Amin was half Kakwa and half Nubian with Sudanese blood. In 1946, he joined the Kings African Rifles. He then went to Britain for officer training at the School of Infantry at Wilshire and to Sterling in Scotland. He took a parachute course in Israel. Amin, who was almost illiterate, had a gift for languages. He knew Lugbara, Kakwa, Luganda, Acholi, and Swahili. He quickly became proficient in English.

Amin was a rugby player and was Ugandan Army heavyweight boxing champion from 1951-1960. The British later commissioned him and when British rule ended in 1963, he held the rank of Captain. He took an advanced paratroopers course in Israel earning high praise from his Israeli instructors.

Amin was a Colonel commanding the army, when in 1966 Uganda was plunged into a bloody internal crisis, in part, the legacy of the constitution given the new country by the departing British. This had set up a federal state, but had granted considerable autonomy to the biggest of four ancient tribal kingdoms within it, especially that of Buganda, under its Kabaka (King).

While the non-Ganda Obote, the goat herder's son from the relatively impoverished North, was the Federal Prime Minister, the Kabaka of Buganda was made president of the Federal Ugandan State.

In 1966, tension between Prime Minister Obote and the Kabaka, Sir Edward Mutesa, erupted into the open. Obote proclaimed himself President, scrapped the ancient kingdoms, and called on Colonel Amin to shell Mengo Hill – the Kabaka capital – and to use his troops to quell Ugandan resistance. In Idi Amin's words, "The streets of Kampala were full of dead bodies."

The Kabaka, a graduate of Britain's exclusive Magdalene College at Cambridge and honorary Colonel in the Grenadier Guards, fled later dying of suspected alcoholic poisoning in England.

Therefore, Obote ruled Uganda in another uneasy alliance – this time with Colonel Amin. In January 1967, Amin rose to the rank of brigadier, with command over all of the country's armed forces, and became a major general the following year. He emerged unscathed from an investigation into allegations that he was involved in illegal gold dealings. He explained that he had been paid large sums of money by revolutionaries in northeastern Zaire (now the Democratic Republic of the Congo) to purchase nonmilitary supplies.

In 1970, Obote and Amin began to fall out. The President reduced the general to the administrative job of Chief of Staff and gave direct control of the army to a brigadier. The increasingly taut alliance finally collapsed in January of 1971, when soldiers of the fifth Malire Mechanised Battalion – mostly men from Amin's own West Nile District – killed their officers and swept the general into the Presidency, while Obote was away in Singapore attending a Commonwealth Prime Minister's Conference.

In exile in neighboring Tanzania where President Nyerere refused to recognize Amin, Obote said to the press that the General had seized power to avert further investigation into his conduct. General Amin claimed that what had actually happened was that soldiers whose loyalty to him had endured, had thwarted a plot by Obote to have him murdered and to display his severed head in front of Kampala's parliament.

In Tanzania, Obote was joined up to two thousand more Ugandan exiles – many of whom were soldiers fleeing from what they said were bloody purges by General Amin's men of troops who belonged to the Acholi and Langi tribes, held to be Obote loyalists. Acholi and Langi soldiers had been hacked to death, shot or clubbed, their exiles reported. After border clashes between Uganda and Tanzania the preceding year, Obote's exiles launched a major guerilla attack across General Amin's southern frontier in September 1972. The general alleged that they were backed by Dr. Nyerere and ordered his planes to bomb Tanzanian towns. His troops crushed the invading force. The exiles died in vicious firefights with the crack, thousand man Simba battalion, and suspected sympathizers were rounded up and taken to Kampala's Makindye Military Prison.

In December 1972, Amin ordered a government takeover of over 40 foreign owned businesses and tea estates, the majority of them British. They included eight of Uganda's biggest firms.

The following May, he announced his government would take over all of the remaining British firms in Uganda thus leading to nationalization.

Before startled guests at a diplomatic reception, Amin personally interrogated one of the leaders of the aborted insurgency – former Information Minister Alex Ojera – who was led in wearing only a pair of khaki trousers with his hands bound behind his back.

With the invasion routed, Somalia helped to negotiate a five-point peace pledge between Tanzania and

Uganda, but President Nyerere made the move towards recognition of Amin as Uganda's Head of State.

Idi Amin took one of his first controversial steps in 1972 when in his "economic war" he expelled some 40,000 Asians holding British passports. A large number were traders, shopkeepers and artisans.

I remember seeing one of the groups of Asians at Entebbe Airport, being herded, like cattle, onto Ugandan Airlines for expulsion. Most of the Indians eventually settled in England. I witnessed gold earrings being torn from the women's ears. One Indian woman lost her ring finger because the soldiers could not remove the ring from it. Amin later said that God had told him in a dream to take this action, at transforming Uganda into a "Black Man's Country".

There were predictions that Uganda would collapse economically. But, despite cuts from western powers, Uganda survived, though plagued with shortages of essential consumer goods and petrol. The pro-Libya Amin sent shock waves through the world with a telegram on the Middle East situation addressed to United Nations Secretary General, Kurt Waldheim, in September of 1972. The telegram, which was also sent to Mrs. Golda Meir, then Israel's Prime Minister, said "Germany was the right place when Hitler was Prime Minister and Supreme Commander". The telegram resulted in the United States suspending a ten million dollar loan to Uganda. On another occasion, Amin was reported as saying that he was disappointed to find, on a visit to Berlin, there was no memorial to Adolf Hitler.

Confronted with torrents of international criticism, the big, broad-shouldered soldier who stands six feet four inches tall and was, for nine years, heavyweight boxing champion in Uganda, appeared totally unruffled completely convinced of the righteousness of his own actions.

He consistently captured world headlines in his first years in power, then for 12 months as chairman of the Organization of African Unity (OAU) from 1975 to 1976. As he relinquished his post, he was a central figure in a hijacked airliner drama at Entebbe airport. A detailed account of this hijacking will appear in the chapter on "The Danger".

He has been vilified in other countries as a dictator (one British political leader called him a "Black Hitler") and a racist. He has been accused of launching a reign of terror in Uganda massacring tens of thousands of political opponents, charged with planning to invade Kenya, and cooperating with hijackers.

Idi Amin Dada customarily wore the blue battle dress of a paratrooper, with a pistol in his belt. He once said, "The only being I fear is God" and he acted that way, appearing to thrive on controversy.

To his critics, President Amin turned a bland smiling face, sometimes denying charges, and sometimes just ignoring them. At times he appeared belligerent one day and conciliatory the next. The conduct of "Big Daddy", as he is sometimes known, was unpredictable. An unlikely combination of severe critics ranged from Daniel Moynihan, former United States Ambassador to the United Nations to Ahmed Sekou Toure, radical President of Guinea.

During his first five years in power, Amin enraged both his neighbors and partners in the East African community of Kenya and Tanzania.

In Kenya, in early 1976, marchers in mass demonstrations carried effigies of the Ugandan leader, which they proceeded to behead and burn. The demonstrations followed a speech in which Amin said he would look into the possibility of claiming major portions of Kenya and the Sudan as historic parts of Uganda.

Tension between Kenya and Uganda reached a new peak in the middle of 1976, with charge and counter-charge. A Kenyan government statement in July 1976 called Amin "The world's greatest dictator of modern times, a Fascist, warmonger, and sadist". A Tanzanian government statement the previous year called him a murderer, oppressor and Black Fascist. In June 1974, the Genevabased International Commission of Jurists declared in a report that Uganda had seen "total breakdown of the rule of law".

Amin dismissed stories of atrocities and disappearances in Uganda. But he once claimed if he had not seized power, Obote would have had him killed and put his head on public display. Tanzania, Botswana, Mozambique and Zambia all stayed away from the OAU summit, which elected Amin OAU Chairman in 1975.

In July 1976, Amin was the center of an international storm arising from the hijack drama at Entebbe airport. Pro-Palestinian guerillas hijacked an Air France airbus and held hostage over a hundred passengers, most of them Israelis. Armed Israeli commandos who swooped down in three planes and flew the passengers back to Israel rescued all but three, who were shot dead. Left behind was Mrs. Dora Bloch, who had been taken to the hospital before the rescue operation.

Amin maintained that before the Israeli commando swoop, he had arranged the release of two batches of hostages totaling 147 people, and was still negotiating for the release of the remaining hundred. But Israeli Defense Minister, Shimon Peres, declared flatly that the Ugandan army had cooperated with the hijackers. He told the Knesset (Israel's Parliament) "This is unprecedented to the best of my knowledge." Britain and Israel both held the Ugandan Government responsible for the disappearance and death of Mrs. Bloch, who had dual citizenship. Although the Israeli operation was a violation of Ugandan territory, it was widely supported in Western countries. Amin, trained as a paratrooper in Israel, broke off diplomatic relations with that country in 1972, expelling all the Israeli nationalists. In return, Colonel Muammar Gaddafi, leader of oil-rich Libya and ardent anti-Zionist, gave Uganda substantial financial aid. Gaddafi remained a firm friend of Amin since that time.

Amin himself said there had been several attempts on his life. One of the most famous happened in June 1976 when grenades were thrown at the Jeep in which he was traveling in Kampala. He was uninjured but his bodyguard was killed.

From time to time, Western experts tried to penetrate the psychology and motivation of Amin. Some suggested he was a simple soldier out of his depths in the sophisticated world of international politics. One assessment came from Dennis Hills, a British lecturer who lived in Uganda for twelve years. He claimed in July 1976, that with all of Amin's bizarre behavior and temperament, Amin had won admiration from his own people and even from some African leaders because he personified aggressive Black national leadership. Hills spent 101 days in Uganda under sentence of death after writing a book in which he described the Ugandan leader as a "village tyrant", a phrase he later retracted as one of the conditions for his release. One clue to the psychology of Idi Amin may come in the way in which he came to sign himself: Alhaji Field Marshall Dr. Idi Amin Dada, VC, DSO, MC. But these initials did not, as a Ugandan spokesman has explained, stand for the famous British military decorations of the Victoria Cross, Distinguished Service Order, and Military Cross. Uganda introduced it's own Victory Cross, Distinguished Service Order and Military Cross, all held by Idi Amin Dada.

Alhaji is the honorific name used by those who have made the pilgrimage to Mecca. Amin, the Muslim, went to Mecca in 1974. The doctorate was an honorary degree – LL.D. (Doctor of Laws) awarded by the Makerere University in Kampala. The University citation gave what can be regarded as official evaluation of Amin's work. It says that within 5 years of coming to power, Idi Amin Dada had become the spokesman for Africa and the ardent champion of the oppressed people of Southern Africa, the Middle East, Southeast Asia, and America. As the chairman of the OAU, he had made Uganda "the pivot of African affairs". It added, "At considerable risk to his life, Field Marshall Amin restored the rights of the people of Uganda over their economic destiny and asserted their political rights in the face of immense imperialist pressures from some big powers."

Idi Amin Dada held the rank of Major General when he carried out the 1971 coupe that unseated Dr. Milton Obote. In July 1975 he acquired the highest military rank, Field Marshall. Uganda radio (Voice of Uganda) announced that the decision to promote him had been taken by a meeting of two thousand officers and men of the Ugandan army, following a meeting of the Defense

Council, ruling body of the military government. In June 1976, the Defense Council announced that Field Marshall Amin had been appointed President for Life. The "economic destiny" phrase evidently referred to Amin's expulsion of the Asians in 1972. Though a considerable embarrassment in Britain, which gave sanctuary to thousands of the displaced citizens, the abrupt action tended to do Amin well, rather than harm, in the eyes of many Africans. This was particularly so in Kenya which has a large and prosperous Asian business and trading community but where official policy encourages the advancement of wananchi (natives). With Britain, the pendulum of Amin's relations swung from warm friendship to coolness, bordering on animosity and back again.

The President once demonstrated his "anti-colonial" stance by driving his new sedan directly across the neatly tended lawns of state house, the official Presidential residence that was once the seat of British Colonial governors. In July 1976, his official radio warned that if any Royal Air Force planes were sited over Uganda, on a mission to take out and repatriate British citizens in Uganda, they would be shot down (Britain denied having any such plans).

Yet the man who learned from British officers how to be a soldier demonstrated many times that he retained a warm regard and admiration for Britain. In December 1973, he said "I have repeatedly stated that we consider the British among our best friends." Inviting Queen Elizabeth to visit Uganda, he said in one telegram that Uganda loved her very much and millions would welcome her if she accepted the invitation.

Relations were always extremely tense with Tanzania. In September 1972, following a series of border incidents, an armed force of Ugandan exiles crossed over from Tanzania intent on unseating Amin. Tanzanian President, Julius Nyerere, called the Ugandan leader a "racist". President Amin sent a telegram to the Tanzanian President saying "I love you very much and if you were a woman I would even consider marrying you, although you have gray hair on your head." This was one of the countless "joker" telegrams sent by Amin to world leaders and widely publicized. In another, he offered to take over from Queen Elizabeth as head of the commonwealth. Such telegrams may have been one factor influencing the New York Times when it described Amin as a "malevolent clown."

One of Amin's actions for which he was most condemned internationally was the murder of the Anglican Archbishop of Uganda, Rwanda, Burungi and Zaire (now the Democratic Republic of the Congo) the Most Reverend Jani Luwum. Reverend Luwum was reported shot dead together with two of Amin's own ministers, who had fallen out of favor with Amin's murder squad, known as the State Research Unit. Official Kampala radio claimed that the three had died in a car crash as a result of their attempt to overpower the soldier who was driving them away for questioning. The murder of Luwum, which took place at the end of 1976, was attributed to Amin's growing antipathy for Christian leaders. It is understood Luwum had never condoned any of his actions. His murder was followed by a period of relative quiet, interrupted only by a few internal skirmishes within the ranks of his mercenary soldiers. The most important of these was the final rift in 1978 between him and his Vice President, which culminated in the Vice President being involved in a near fatal car crash. This was indeed the beginning of the end for Idi Amin Dada. For the split between loyal soldiers – mostly from his Kakwa tribe – and mercenaries was quite fundamental. It was to draw public attention away from the fighting between the two factions that he invaded Tanzania at the end of last year and occupied huge chunks of territory. These reasons were kept quiet to the Ugandans and they were told that the reason for the invasion of Tanzania was because they were stealing the metal roofs from the people's houses. Tanzania's counter attack was coupled with a new determination by exiled factions to unite and topple "the snake" in Kampala. This onslaught on Amin never relented.

Government sources said that they believed Amin left in a Libyan airliner in April of 1979 headed for Tripoli. News and eyewitness reports said that he had probably fled to northern Uganda from his last known stronghold in the industrial city of Jinja, east of Kampala. Sudanese news and official reports said that Amin would land there, refuel and then continue on to Libya or Iraq where his family was living. Amin as we know eventually landed in Libya, was expelled from there, and went to Saudi Arabia and finally left for the Democratic Republic of the Congo in an attempt to return to Uganda. He never reached Uganda. He died in 2003 at 80 years of age. This was a man who had brutalized and terrorized his nation for a decade and was left to justice by nature. He was never brought to trial and was never executed.

Politics is, as we know the use of power, authority, and influence. Power is the ability to bring about results often through the possession or use of forceful means.

Power is backed up by the potential use of force. It exists in relation to others. In Uganda, the tribe is the unit of power. They are now in the process of democratization and this refers to the process of transformation from an authoritarian regime to one that is democratic. This process includes several features – the end of torture, the liberation of political prisoners, the lifting of censorship, and the toleration of some opposition. A military commission headed by Paulo Muwanga took power in May 1980 and subsequently organized general elections in December of the same year. Milton Obote became President for the second time after rigging the general elections. Under his rule, a lot of human rights violations were committed and his army ruthlessly murdered thousands of Ugandans. In July 1985, Obote was deposed by his own army. A Military Council under the Chairmanship of General Tito Okello replaced him. Okello's military junta also continued committing human rights atrocities until the National Resistance Army (NRA), military wing of the National Resistance Movement (NRM) in January 1986, removed it.

Under the leadership of the current President Yoweri K. Museveni, the National Resistance Army opposed the coming to power of Obote through rigged elections. The NRA, therefore, fought a protracted people's war from 1981 until decisive victory in January 1986. Following the takeover of power, the NRM immediately formed a broad-based government and moved swiftly to re- establish law and order all over the country.

Amin was married five times and is estimated to have had about 200 children. It is difficult to keep track of them. Every now and then he would announce that he had fathered a child by a woman that no one had ever heard of before. He divorced three of his first four wives, keeping one named Medina. He then married Sarah, known flippantly as "Suicide Sarah" because she was a member of the Ugandan mechanized so- called Suicide Regiment at the time of her marriage to Amin in July 1975. This was the time of the OAU Kampala Summit.

His near one-decade of absolute power was marked by brutality and buffoonery that have left him with the tragic-comic image of a national leader who combines the ruthlessness of a Genghis Khan with the belly laughs of a Charlie Chaplin. Since seizing power in 1971, he conducted a reign of terror against his own people and foreigners living in the country that is estimated to have left at least 300,000 people dead --a figure comparable to the population of Nairobi.

The man he deposed, President Milton Obote, once described him as "The Greatest Brute an African mother has ever brought to life". He reduced the nation's economy to a shambles largely as a result of the expulsion of Asian traders, who formed the backbone of the nation's entrepreneurial life, and purged the bureaucracy of thousands of educated Ugandans whose talents were badly needed in the largely illiterate country. They sought refuge abroad.

The Work

Have you ever had a job that you loved so much that you literally ran to work every morning? The climate was perfect in the foothills of the Mountains of the Moon (Rwenzori Mountains) some 6,000 feet above sea level. Temperature in the early morning is about 60 degrees and goes to nearly 90 degrees at noon without any humidity. In the evenings the light of the sun comes to a very sudden darkness because we are located on the equator.

The small town, Fort Portal, had a Catholic hospital called Virika. It was here that I worked as a Secretary-Accountant, trying to get the hospital out of debt. Too much free service was being given to the discharged patients. Vietnamese, Korean, Chinese, American, Russian, Algerians, Egyptians and Ugandan doctors worked together with the African staff to give good care to patients who were Africans as well as Europeans. My days were filled with learning the language and the culture, as well as routing through the financial crisis. The cost of treating typhoid, smallpox, T.B., elephantisis, bilharzia, and the various anemias especially hookworm anemia as well as other exotic diseases took its toll on me. Seeing the flaccid rash of measles on a malnourished child ran through my brain every night.

Witnessing the attempts to save the lives of children with measles, I became familiar with a procedure called clysis. This procedure was used as a last ditch effort to save children whose veins had collapsed in shock and the only access for giving the I.V. fluids for rehydration was directly into the abdomen. Many of these children survived.

Maternal and Neonatal Tetanus has been eliminated in most developed countries as a Public Health threat. Yearly 180,000 infants and 30,000 mothers die of MNT (Maternal Neonatal Tetanus) in Africa. The U.S. Fund for UNICEF, coupled with other non-profit organizations, are leading healthcare to eliminate MNT. Tetanus Toxoid vaccine is now distributed to the mothers as a Uniject device (TIME Magazine).

The ecological fate of Uganda lies with the elimination of malaria. Malaria kills 2 million African children each year. Malaria zaps worker productivity, scares away many businesses, and decreases population growth. Instead of having 2 to 3 children, the Ugandans choose to have 6 to 7 children to ensure the longevity of their family and tribe. We found that the treatment of malaria was necessary; but, realizing the transient climate, the specific types of mosquitoes, and the breeding sites are all factors. Medications cost a little over a dollar per treatment.

I remember as if it were yesterday, my first malarial attack. I was feeling very feverish; but went on duty anyhow. I later went to the lab and had a malaria smear done at the height of my fever. The doctor placed me on Cloraquin for malaria. At that time, it was taken for two weeks. I could hardly open my eyes, as I was so photophobic. I had been bitten by *the falciparium*

Malariae mosquito and would have many symptoms – diarrhea, shivers, fever, and malaise. Sometimes I had all the symptoms together; other times a combination.

One of the diseases that I noticed that was being treated repeatedly in our hospital was hookworm anemia. In an article by Dr. Musisi, Assistant Director of Medical Services under the Ministry of Health in Entebbe, he stated that in Uganda the influence and customs (social cultural behavior and beliefs) in promoting diseases has had very little exploration, although if thoroughly studied solutions may be found to control or even eradicate many of our endemic diseases. Hookworm infection and disease in the varied tribal societies in Uganda is rampant. Man is the only host for this parasite and is, therefore, himself alone to blame for its existence and wide spread. The hookworm enters the host through the bare feet and hand to mouth contamination is assured.

Throughout Uganda not a single hospital can claim to be free of continually treating multiple victims of this parasite. In worst areas, one medical doctor observer claimed incidence to be as high as 80 percent in the population around his hospital. On the other hand, campaigns to advise the public to build and to use latrines started many years in the past. It has had further momentum in the late sixties when the Home and Environmental Competitions were introduced. It is therefore, striking to note, that these many years of vigorous campaigns have not reduced the incidence of this parasitic infection. In fact, in rural areas even in homes where latrines do exist, hookworm disease is still a burden to the members of the families. There must be other factors that are causing this artificial vicious circle. These are the social cultural factors. A few of these factors that I have been able to unearth in a little survey during the 1970's are important in public health nursing.

Children are very precious; in fact a woman without a child in Africa feels inadequate. Children are valued differently in many tribal societies; they are assets for earning a living for a family. At a very early age they look after flocks of goats, sheep and herds of cattle. Some are responsible for maintaining large shambas (simple housing) as well as harvesting crops. If they are girls, once they are mature and ready for marriage, they are literally bought by prospective husbands with large sums of money or many herds of cattle. A woman in a family during her childbearing years is very precious as a potential source of capital. There are beliefs and behaviors in some tribes valued as methods of preventing infertility in a woman. They are not allowed to use latrines for fear of causing sterility or sometimes for fear of reducing their sexual arousal.

When they are pregnant, this is where they are strictly forbidden from using latrines for fear of the fetus popping out and falling into the pit. Others believe that by using latrines by a heavy mother leads to brain damage or seizures in a child before birth. And for the fear of cross infections, there is also an objection to accumulating the feces in the pits that diseases will cross from those infected to those who are free from infection.

When children are born, they must also be protected. In some areas, children's feces must not be deposited in the pit until the child is able to walk and talk. Depositing feces in the pit is believed to retard the child's mental development at an early age. During this period, the feces are deposited on a banana plant (Nakabululu) to hasten the child's physical and mental ability. It is also feared that a child may fall into the pit and die. In other areas, parents are shy to be found going into latrines by their children, hence, children must use gardens or other grounds.

In many tribes, in-laws are treated with great respect and delicacy and hence their hosts never closely accept them. There are beliefs that close association with them leads to tremors, body swelling, and depigmentation diseases. To avoid this calamity, they never share latrines with their hosts; instead they are obliged to find convenient places. Tribes consist of herdsmen and are migratory in search of grass and water for their animals especially during dry season. This group without permanent homes is accustomed to stooling in the bushes and the use of a latrine is almost unknown and unacceptable to them. On some lakeshores, the soil is sandy with a low water table, so fishermen in these villages, through environmental influences are not accustomed to using latrines. Latrines cannot be built on sandy areas where water is near the surface; they hence find bushes convenient to hold and hide their feces.

These social cultural beliefs and behaviors are continuing to promote the existence and spread of hookworm anemia disease despite the efforts to eradicate it. A drive to cause a change in beliefs and to value health practice will be the main tool of success.

There must be collaboration between doctors working in hospitals and public health staff working in the field. The latter will be struck to find a child, mother or father admitted and being transfused with inferon or blood while, in the home, there is a well-finished latrine. Such cases are many and quite common, that pass unnoticed by health staff because they never visit the hospital wards. It is strongly advocated that they should start making routine visits to wards and observe from disease spectrum the successes and failures of their work not in terms of structural successes and figures alone, but also in terms of falling instances of preventable diseases.

Uganda has been one of the leading nations among developing countries in the field of nutrition science and research. The presence of the Medical Research Councils' nutrition unit since the early 1950's to the early 1970's gave an added impetus to many nutritional activities in the country. Many papers by Uganda-based research workers have been published in international journals or presented at international conferences, some of which have taken place in Uganda. The interest taken by many international bodies such as the World Health Organization, the Food and Agricultural Organization, the United Nations Children's Fund, World Food Program, Save the Children's Fund, Oxfam, and many others have also stimulated a lot of thinking about nutrition.

There is a policy that has been formulated in the different Five Year Development Plans and now the Action Program (1977-1981). These activities are: (a) increase food and cash crops production, the latter aimed at raising foreign exchange to buy the foods that Uganda cannot produce, (b) the Youth Development Schemes such as the Namutamba Project, the Youth Settlement Schemes and the Young Farmers of Uganda, (c) the Inter-provincial Home and Environment Competitions, (d) various nutritional rehabilitation schemes such as the Mwanamugimu, originally sponsored by the Save the Children's Fund, now fully run by the Ministry of Health; the UNICEF supported nutrition scouts pilot project at Kayunga, soon to become the basis of the Primary

Healthcare Pilot Project, (e) the Maternal and Child Health activities of the Ministry of Health, (f) community development activities such as Women's Clubs, Youth Clubs, etc., (g) the Ministry of Education activities such as school meals and health education activities at school, and the teaching of agriculture.

While I was in Fort Portal, the bills for the various treatments of hospitalization would come across my desk daily. I found the charges and collection of the money for these services could not compare with the actual bedside treatment of our patients. I grew discontented every day with my job as a secretary-accountant and longed to go to nursing and midwifery school. I wanted action and did I ever get it!

I remember talking to Dr. S. Okware, MOH Epidemiologist, about "The Importance of Venereal Disease Decree". Dr. Okware stated that his Excellency Life President Idi Amin, who is currently holding the portfolio of the Minister of Health, signed the Venereal Disease Decree whose main emphasis is on the systemic prevention and control of venereal disease. The Decree for all intents and purposes would curb the general increase incidence of venereal disease in Uganda.

The Decree clearly calls for a multidisciplinary effort, not only for health personnel but also for the tribal chiefs, police, etc., if this disgraceful malady is to be contained in Uganda. In short, it demands teamwork from everyone who is in a position to assist. This eliminates the incarceration of the people with venereal disease.

Food and nutrition were always a high priority in all of the hospitals in Uganda. Dr. J. Kakitahi, lecturer in Makerere Institute of Public Health, presented a paper at the WHO Regional Committee for Africa held in

Brazzaville in September 1977. He stated that Uganda has a population of about 20 million people, depending mainly on subsistence farming. Sixty-eight percent of the population at this time includes children under fifteen and women of the reproductive age (15-45 years). It is this portion that constitutes Uganda's priority public health nutrition problem.

Studies have shown that almost all of the children, particularly those in rural areas, go through a period of marginal under-nutrition or delayed growth during early childhood. School meals have also deteriorated, proving to be inadequate and resulting in poor growth and development as well as poor school performance. Such nutritional problems have been attributed mainly to the climatic conditions, ethnic groupings and their associated cultural and food attitudes and economic traditions, all of which have been noted as determinants of food growth and what is consumed in a given area.

Current activities are based on a comprehensive and integrated approach involving other relevant Ministries particularly Agriculture, Community Development, Education, and Finance. These activities are geared to preventing malnutrition of all grades. This is carried out at hospital units, during home visiting, or during school health examinations. The rehabilitation process does not include dietary aspects only, but social, environmental, cultural and all other aspects that affect the nutritional status of those at risk. The same process continues into the community when they are discharged from hospitals. This is done mainly through regular home visiting and specific visits to problem homes.

The ultimate aim of all of these activities coupled with health education is to change people's eating patterns and attitudes, so as to improve on the quality and quantity of the foods produced and consumed. Other public health activities like general immunization, improvement of environmental sanitation, water supply and wider coverage of health education, that have been found to contribute to the improvement of nutritional status, continued to be encouraged daily. The government is working out a well-defined policy to fight malnutrition in all of its forms and for all ages. Uganda set up a "Nutritional Council" including the Ministry of Health and other departments, to plan, execute, and coordinate nutritional activities within a set policy of economical and social development. The Government has built health centers in rural areas with the aim of having at least a health center for every 20,000 people.

All of these educational ideas filled my heart and mind, and with the help of Mrs. Lucy Walusimbi, I returned to the United States and went to a nursing program at Philadelphia General Hospital and four years later I went to England to complete an eighteen-month course in midwifery. I then returned to Jinja Hospital to help set up the first Post-Graduate Pediatric Program for Uganda Registered Nurses.

The Jinja Hospital staff always commented on how they thought some of the measles vaccine was not effective. We studied the problem as a research project and found the importance of the Cold Chain Maintenance.

Dr. Stanley Sendaula Kasumba, administrator of public health, authored a paper that helped us greatly in solving our problem. Measles is one of the four infectious causes of infant mortality along with gastroenteritis, bronchopneumonia and malaria. The disease can be effectively controlled with measles vaccine immunization, if the ideal conditions for handling the vaccine are meticulously observed.

Measles vaccine is produced by growing a weakened measles virus in tissue culture (cells obtained from the embryos of fertilized hens eggs at a temperature of 34 degrees centigrade). The virus grown in the cells is spilled out into the liquid medium, separated from the cells and freeze-dried immediately. The virus is very sensitive to heat and light and has to be handled with great care. Refrigeration is essential, Cold Chain Maintenance, from the time it leaves the factory, through the various stages of its handling until it finally gets inoculated into the child.

After clearing the vaccine from the airport on arrival, it goes directly to the Central Medical Stores for storage without delay, and placed in the correct freezer, refrigerator or cold rooms at a temperature of 2 to 4 degrees centigrade. Medium-size isothermic boxes containing ice are used to transport the vaccine from the Central Medical Stores to the peripheral centers in the districts, where it should be kept in the refrigerators at the ideal range of temperatures. In every container an unbreakable thermometer is kept for checking on the temperature so as to insure the effectiveness of the refrigeration chain.

In a nutshell, handling of the measles vaccine requires that the cold chain system be ideally maintained at every stage of the vaccine's life from the time it leaves the factory until it gets injected into the child. If this is not done, the vaccine loses potency and the protection it is intended to give when it is injected becomes lost, with the resultant adverse consequences together with the loss of faith in the efficiency of the vaccination scheme on the part of the parents.

The government learned its lessons the hard way. They learned never to give the vaccine to a child who was suffering from kwashiorkor, allergic conditions, or when the child is febrile.

Over and over again daily we had shortages of one thing after another. The only thing that was not in short supply was cases of measles and other life threatening diseases. Often we would have no medications – the only antibiotic in the country may have been gentamycin. I could not change the people themselves or their culture. Nor did I want to. I wanted to change their way of thinking about sterility and cleanliness.

One of the most upsetting practices I found when I worked at Jinja Hospital was that the nurses washed the rubber gloves and dried them in the sun. They then turned them inside out, powdered them, and placed the gloves in a metal drum to be sterilized in the Central Supply autoclave. Here in America, sterile gloves are an integral purchase by every hospital and are disposable. As a regular practice, we used to wear three pairs of gloves during a delivery. And yet, years later, one of my Post-Graduate Pediatric students died from AIDS as a result of a needle stick from an AIDS positive patient.

One of the most debilitating shortages was the disconnection of electricity due to "no spare parts" for the Jinja Dam. I would often be in the delivery room and the light would go out. We would always keep the equipment in the same position so that when we had no electricity and before the backup generator would kick in, we would know how to proceed with the infant's delivery. I remember very vividly one delivery like this when the baby's head was felt. The lights went out and I told the father of the baby to strike a match. He followed his instructions very carefully and a beautiful baby boy was born. The family named the baby "Deo Gracias Ekibiritti" which means "Thank God We Had Matches".

In America, however, there are no shortages of medical supplies and sophisticated diagnostic technology. But sometimes the best diagnostic tools are the most natural. In Uganda, sometimes the child's symptoms were very obvious to the mother. In nursing, we always teach the students the importance of listening to the patient and the mother, as the clues are usually right in front of us. A mother came to the clinic with her infant and stated that he tasted salty. I asked my students how the mother knew this and they said that she had probably licked him while showing affection. By stating this, the mother gave the biggest clue of all to help the doctors with their diagnosis. The infant had cystic fibrosis. Even in the absence of technology, these simple village people have come up with their own effective methods of diagnosis.

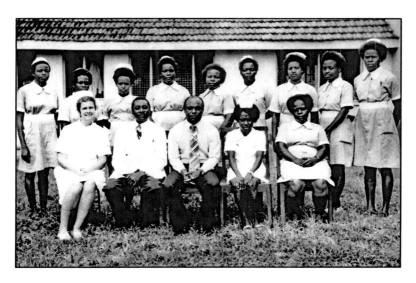

The official photo of Jinja Hospital's first Post-Graduate Pediatric
Class. Mary Hale is in the front row first on the left.

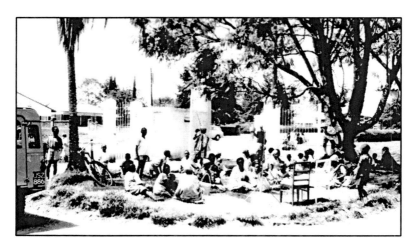

Front gate at Virika Hospital in Fort Portal, Uganda.
Daily gathering of Mother's Teaching Class.

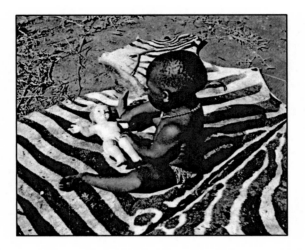

This picture tells the story of why I went to Uganda, East Africa - to help the children who could not help themselves.

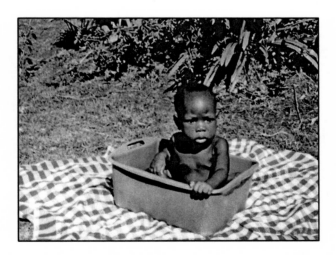

Stella Maris was found in the gutter on a main street in Jinja. She was breastfeeding and her Mother had died. She is now a pediatrician at the hospital where she was raised.

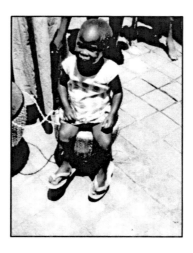

Local child in Fort Portal Market sitting on a drum.
Note the large flip-flops, which she will grow into.

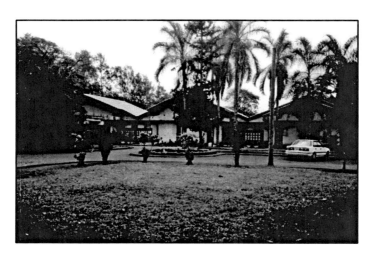

Jinja Hospital Children's Ward given to us by President Idi Amin.
Located a mile from main hospital.

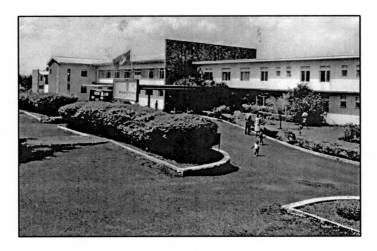

The Crested Crane Hotel in Jinja, Uganda,
where I stayed for six months of my contract.

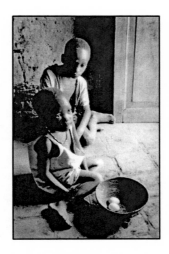

Payment of a hospital bill at Fort Portal, Uganda.

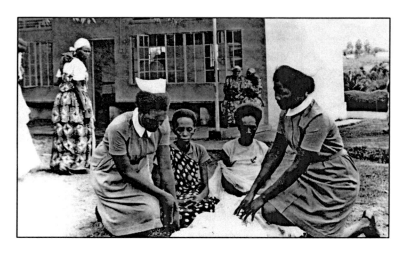

CPR Training in front garden of Virika Hospital
at Fort Portal, Uganda.

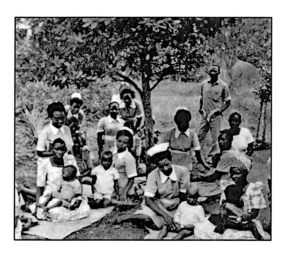

Post-Graduate Nursing students with Mothers and patients at
"Mwanamugimu" (translation "you have fallen into good things")
nutritional garden.

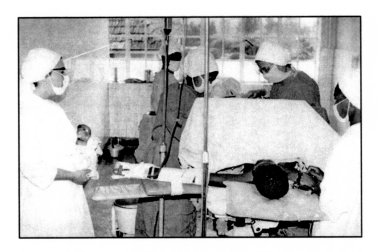

These physicians were from India and Yugoslavia. Others were from U.S.A., England, China, Vietnam, Egypt, Brazil, and Pakistan.

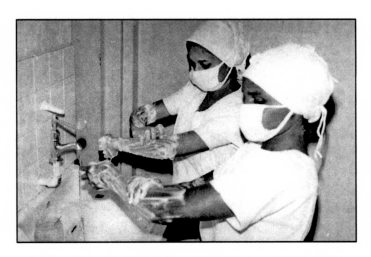

Cleanliness and sterility were emphasized as something that could not be compromised.

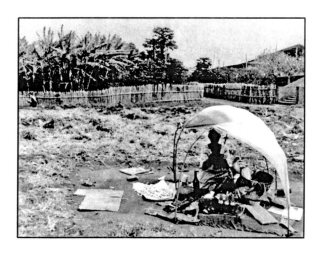

The local coca-cola store across the street from
Virika Hospital, Fort Portal, Uganda.

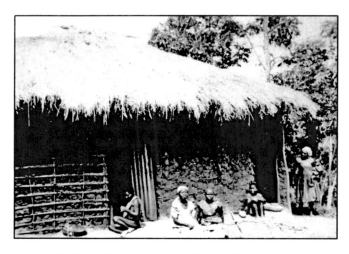

A shamba in the village near Fort Portal, Uganda, East Africa.

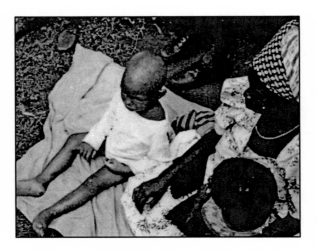

A typical child with kwashiokor and marasmus.
Note the edema and loss of hair.

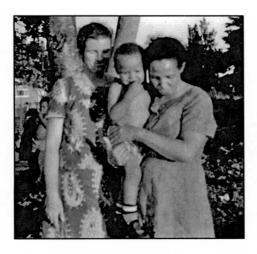

Mary Hale, Julianna's son Robert, and Julianna.

The Danger

"The Entebbe Rescue Mission" serves as an instructional experience to our U.S. Marine Corps, even today.

The Israel Defense Forces released the facts about this one time lesson for us. I was working at Jinja Hospital, when my machine-gunned luggage arrived from Entebbe International Airport some six months after my arrival from furlough. The shampoo plastic bottles were leaking all over my bullet-ridden uniforms and other clothes.

What exactly happened during the raid on Entebbe? The hijackers were five members of the Popular Front for the Liberation of Palestine and two German terrorists. Uganda ruler, Idi Amin, was open and receptive to helping the terrorist cause. Ugandan soldiers held over 250 passengers and crew hostage at Entebbe Airport. The hostages were eventually segregated into two groups: non-Jews and Jews/Israelis.

On June 27, 1976 four terrorists forced an Air France Airbus to land in Uganda in the heart of distant Africa. They quickly demanded that Israel release 53 convicted terrorists held elsewhere. The hijackers freed the French crew and non-Jewish passengers while retaining 105

Jewish and Israeli hostages. A forty-eight hour deadline was set before executions would begin.

Faced with little choice, the Israeli government announced that it would enter into negotiations. This bought the precious time needed to consolidate a seemingly impossible military option. A new ultimatum was issued for 13:00 hours on Sunday, July 4th. The only airplane capable of this rescue operation was the C130 Hercules. On July 1, the mission's overall commander, Brigadier General Dan Shomron (later to become Israel Defense Forces Chief of Staff), presented his plan to the IDF Commander and Israel's Defense Minister. The next day they all witnessed a full-scale dress rehearsal. The incredible rescue was deemed possible.

Shomron's plan was based on several advantages that the Israelis had over the terrorists. The Entebbe Airport, at which the hostages were being held, was built by an Israeli construction firm that was able to provide Shomron with blueprints. Moreover, the released non-Jewish hostages, were able to describe the terrorists, their arms, and their positioning. As a result of this information, the IDF decided to send in an overwhelmingly powerful force – over 200 of the best soldiers the army had to offer participated in the raid, all of them heavily armed.

Finally, the element of surprise was probably the biggest edge that Israel held. According to Shomron: "You had more than a hundred people sitting in a small room, surrounded by terrorists with their finger on the trigger. They could fire in a fraction of a second. We had to fly seven hours, land safely, drive to the terminal area where the hostages were being held, get inside, and eliminate all of the terrorists before any of them could fire." The fact that no one expected the Israelis to take such risks was precisely the reason they took them.

The aircraft took off at 13:20 hours on July 3rd and headed south. Only then was the plan revealed to the Israeli Cabinet, which decided to let the operation continue. The lead Hercules carried the rescue force led by Lt. Colonel Yonatan Netanyahu (the brother of former Prime Minister of Benjamin Netanyahu). It also held two jeeps and the now famous black Mercedes, a perfect copy of Dictator Idi Amin's personal car. Two additional Hercules carried reinforcements and troops assigned to carry out special missions, such as destroying Migs (Russian aircraft) parked nearby. A fourth Hercules was sent to evacuate the hostages. The air package also included two Boeing 707's. One acted as a forward command post. The second, outfitted as an airborne hospital, landed in nearby Nairobi, Kenya. The Hercules was escorted by F4 Phantoms as far as possible – about one third the distance.

Skirting thunderstorms over Lake Victoria, the Hercules transports neared the end of the seven hour forty minute flight. A surprise awaited them: the runway lights were on! Despite this they landed undetected at 23:01 hours (local time) only one minute past their planned arrival time.

The soldiers freed the hostages in a lightning attack killing all eight terrorists in the process. Tragically, force commander Yoni Netanyahu was killed as he led the hostages toward the safety of the aircraft. It was rumored after the raid that the Ugandans at Entebbe airport had played a recording of an infant crying and the force commander turned towards the recording of the infant crying and was shot dead. Additionally, two hostages were killed in the crossfire inside the airport. The other squads accomplished their missions in nearly the same time as the "dry run". By 23:59 hours the planes were on their way home. The operation, which was predicted to last one hour, in fact took only 58 minutes.

One of the Israeli passengers, Mrs. Dora Bloch, was a casualty that was seen by my exchange-nursing students at Mulago Hospital. Mrs. Bloch was showing symptoms of either a choking episode or a heart attack as she sat with the other captives at the Entebbe International Airport.

She was immediately separated from the group and shipped to Mulago Hospital, where she was treated and kept as an inpatient. My students did not give her direct care but would visit her to help with her anxiety.

One night members of the State Research Bureau visited her and closed the door to her hospital room. My students said they heard noises in the hallway and then the door was opened very suddenly. They saw the State Research men dragging Mrs. Bloch and pulling her down the exit stairs. Gunfire was heard and the students scattered – only to be given immediate leave by hospital administrators to go and hide in their villages. The State Research people drove her body to the Mabiru Forrest, where her body was burnt and buried in an unmarked grave.

Mrs. Bloch's personal effects were kept at Mulago Hospital. Her son claimed them five years later. At this time, one of the local villagers who lived near the Mabiru Forrest led him to his mother's unmarked grave and together they dug up Mrs. Block's body, which was returned to Israel for proper burial.

The mission struck a blow at international terrorism. "It resonated far and wide", Shomron later commented. "It showed that you could counter terrorism and that it was worth cooperating to do so." As America celebrated its Bicentennial, the world was reminded that freedom was a value that must be fought for in every generation.

Around this time, there was a U.S. embargo on Ugandan coffee. The Voice of Uganda, the local radio station, announced that Amin wanted to show friendship to the 212 Americans working in Uganda. The date was fixed and we were to meet at the Kampala International Hotel. The night before the meeting, it was cancelled over The Voice of Uganda.

At this time we had no American Embassy in Uganda. The closest embassy was in Nairobi, Kenya. The West German embassy represented the Americans in Uganda. The U. S. citizens would meet with the West German Ambassador under the disguise of a New Year's Eve party, etc. We knew there was a spy planted by them in the Uganda Parliament.

The Voice of Uganda announced another date set for the friendship party. This time it was to be at the Lake Victoria Hotel in Entebbe close to the airport. Then, all of the sudden, that date was cancelled and we were told by Amin to return to our usual duties. We were called to attend a New Year's Eve party with the representatives of the West German government. When we gathered at the Kampala International Hotel, we were told that the spy on the Ugandan Parliament had found out the reason for the cancellation of Amin's friendship party. The spy had said that when the Americans met at the Lake Victoria Hotel at Entebbe, we were going to be thanked for our work in

Uganda and then herded onto a Uganda Airlines airplane and kidnapped to the Sudan.

We found out later when all of us had eventually returned to our country (USA) that our U.S. President had warned Amin with a short message via a diplomatic courier, "…not to touch the hair of one American as U.S. Marines were off the coast of Dar Es Salam, preparing to invade Uganda."

Muammar al-Quaddafi, the Dictator of Libya for the last 38 years, advised Amin not to go through with the kidnapping. He has been a conspicuous enemy of the U.S.

As we worked at Jinja Hospital, the staff would report daily disappearances usually attributed to "car crashes". These disappearances consisted of local farmers, hospital staff, local politicians, and some religious leaders.

As our first Pediatric Post-Graduate students were nearing graduation, I traveled by a small plane all over Uganda to check out the areas in which they would be posted in the service of the Ministry of Health. I wanted to see the areas to which they would be posted to see what they would be experiencing, so that we could instruct them in whatever deficits they had in their courses.

As an example, we taught them not to build hospitals with flat roofs, which always held water and leaked. They were taught to build slanted roofs and placement of the rain barrels to catch the precious rainwater. In the dry season, this water would be welcome.

The plane was very small and I was one of several passengers. The pilot would slide a cooler down the center aisle and told us to help ourselves to Fanta or Coke.

Landing in Arua we gently touched down on a grass airfield with a small building for cover while we waited for our return flight. On one of these return flights to Entebbe, there were 5 Americans who were waiting in this building for the return flight. I started a conversation with them and found out they were mercenaries installing spy satellites for Amin. Who knows what problems this would cause?

The State Research Intelligence Network paralyzed the civilian population with fear. The Asians and other groups controlling most of Ugandan commerce and trade were being expelled as Amin nationalized their properties. There was no common cultural heritage within Uganda.

Most of the candidates for the State Research -- candidates for spying within Uganda -- were sent to Russia for training. The Soviet Union sent them back as "untrainable". The General Service Prison at Nakassero was the location for prisoners who were being interrogated and tortured. The public would walk by the prison and feared the screams of their fellow Ugandans.

On the day I went to Kampala for my expatriate supplies of sugar, cooking oil, soap, and sometimes toilet paper, I heard rumors of an execution in Kampala scheduled for that day. As we turned a corner, we saw men hooded and circled around the clock tower. Their wives and children were all watching for the death of their loved one. The machine guns fired, blood splattered and we scattered only to be haunted for years by the sights and sounds of that day. It was rumored the reason they were executed was that they were not Muslim and would not change their religion.

The State Research followed me during my duties at Jinja Hospital. They used to burst into my room at the Nurses Hostel to see if I was transmitting to London or America. I had a small silver radio, used to keep me sane, as I listened to the BBC or Voice of America. Everything was censored in Uganda. You never complained in public about anything in Uganda. You were cautious, as to whom you would share any of your opinions. The price of an airmail stamp was prohibitive (approximately one month's salary) to write news abroad so no one ever wrote air letters.

My mail was always opened and read and resealed with tape. One day I received a box retaped. The box had contained chocolates, which had been eaten, but the candy papers were intact. There was also a pair of woolen socks, which were intact. One of the air letter forms containing a new crisp ten-dollar American bill, sent by my father, to get butter and Philadelphia Cream Cheese did get through to me. The next one sent a month later did not. The air letter was received, taped closed, and the ten-dollar bill was missing in action! The White Fathers used to take the foreign money to Kenya where they would buy the butter and Philadelphia Cream Cheese and bring it back to me over the border to Uganda. The Philadelphia Cream cheese was such a treat that I would only take a small portion for my bread every day. Although it was kept in my small refrigerator a small pink streak appeared in the center of the cheese. I knew that this was very dangerous; but I continued to eat the cheese after I had removed the pink culture. As a result I got extremely ill with food poisoning. Always being a risk taker, and realizing the preciousness of the cheese, I had eaten the remainder of the cheese which was my downfall.

The "executive" of Obote and Amin led to the disintegration of this whole civilization and culture. The principal areas of the Kingdom regions, judiciary, legislative, executive, and the civil service (kingdoms were forbidden to have local armies and police) were all African-manned and run, with the age-old ability and experience in governing and in the exercise of power. The consequences of imposing an alien system on Uganda were catastrophic, both politically and socially.

The fundamental conflict between the Central Government (the colonial state) and the Non-Colonial State came to a head in a conflict between dictatorship and democracy. In summary, monarchies and the regimes were crushed in 1966 and 1967 by Obote's coups d'état. The policy of the British to build a state of Uganda based on force and deception was continued by the African political leadership under both Obote and Amin, which led eventually to the state itself disintegrating and to the whole civilization and culture being dismantled.

Sometimes it takes a little reflection on symbols to see what is missing in our lives. Uganda's flag was adapted in 1962. According to the Ugandan Tourist Website, "The black colored stripes identified Uganda as a black nation in Africa. The yellow stripes represent the sunshine Uganda enjoys being situated on the equator and the red stripes represent Uganda's brotherhood with the rest of Africa and the world. The crested crane, the national bird of Uganda, remains in the center of the flag and stands on one leg facing the flagpole. The raised leg symbolized that Uganda is not stationary but moving forward. The crane's plumage contains the colors of Uganda's flag and is friendly, gentle and a peace loving bird, characteristics which are true of the Ugandan people. The motto "For God and My Country" reflects upon Uganda as a nation of people who fear God and love their country."

The Ugandans' feelings of disappointment and impatience are understandable. But their sentiments are not a responsible basis for policy. Can tyranny be replaced by the forces of liberty?

The Stories

Children can be a joy to us when they are well. One nine year old getting well to go home, said to me "Your smile is stopped by your ears." It is all in how they perceive life.

The Earthquake
The year of the earthquake was 1966. I lay in bed, as the building shook back and forth. We ran outside – only to see the old cathedral, across the street, in ruins.

After assessing the damage to the hospital and the various casualties, we loaded the Land Rover with sacks of porridge (corn or maize flour) and blankets and headed for an area called Bwamba, which had the most damage. As we arrived in Bwamba, we saw the Bakanjo people coping as best they could. We saw hundreds of displaced people climbing out of the huge cracks in the earth, where they and their houses were swallowed up. For many of them, the only white people they had ever seen were the White Fathers, who ran the local mission.

They ran up to us banging on the car windows to have their pictures taken for money. The women would have skirts of African design, necklaces of bright beads and usually bones in their nose and earlobes. The men simply wore loincloths and bones in their hair. Some of the Ugandan tribes believed that their spirit went into the camera; obviously this tribe did not.

The year of the earthquake, 1966, was called Musisi which meant earthquake. All of the children born in that year assumed the last name of Musisi so later in their life, when they came to the hospital; we all knew the year of their birth.

In Uganda last names are not family-specific. For example: Paulo Musisi was born in 1966; Baraza Muganda was a Ugandan born on a Monday. Both may be from the same family and of course, Deo Gratias Ekibiritti meant, "Thank God we had matches", when the baby was born.

The people who were displaced during the earthquake stayed at the local mission or with their extended families. They would be back in their mud huts within the month and resumed their fishing, hunting, or farming to feed their families.

Outfitting the Ward

When I first toured the Maternity Unit at Jinja Hospital, I noticed they had two incubators and I began to change my opinion of the Neonatal Unit. Once I started working, I found out that the incubators had been donated by Great Britain many years previously. As I investigated their maintenance, I found out that although they looked clean and maintained a therapeutic temperature they never changed the water for humidity. We decided to throw them out, as they were a source for potential infection.

The linens and equipment were desperately in need of replacement. As usual there was no money in the budget. My students told me that if I went to the various companies in the trade district, they felt I could get plenty of donations. They stated that the local merchants would donate to a Muzungu (the white one), who would not sell their goods on the Black Market.

I started my project at the local sugar refinery. That is where I met my best friend, Helen Wagabaza, who was a secretary there. She made sure I got a great donation of sugar to be used at the hospital for the children's porridge. Without their sugar, they would not drink their tea or eat their porridge for breakfast.

Then I went to the lumberyard, the Jinja cotton factory, and various other firms that could supply what we could use in our nursery. They donated cloth for the infants' sheets and diapers, canvas for the hanging cots, wood, foam and plastic covers for the makeshift mattresses.

The hospital sewing room went to work and in a month we had a brand new nursery. We would open one window in the nursery and let in the heat and sunlight; at night we had a donated wall heater.

Each infant cot was a canvas hung on a metal frame. Blue and pink sheets were on top of a plastic covered piece of foam on a wooden board. But I loved most of all the little mosquito nets trimmed with the color of the sheets.

Boiled Cow's Milk

Many of the infants were premature and had to be tube fed. We had a roll of plastic tubing, boiled a small piece and passed it into the infant's stomach. A metal Luer-Lock needle was placed at the end and connected to a syringe.

During the time of infant rapid growth, we would syringe feed with boiled cow's milk. The delivery of a large can of cow's milk would arrive a little past noon each day. The can would be attached to a bicycle and driver for a six-mile journey into the hospital. All the time the tin was in the noon sun. Depending on the cyclist's activities, the milk arrived sour or not sour. We found that the man was having an affair along the roadside on the way to the hospital. All the while the can was in the sun.

Needless to say, we could not use sour milk. One of the staff had said that she used the boiled rice water to help feed her infant many years previously. We tried this and it worked. The infant's diet consisted of boiled cow's milk, sometimes boiled rice water, but never formula.

The care and preparation of foreign formula led to an increase of gastroenteritis and weight loss that often resulted in death. We encouraged breastfeeding. Mother's breast milk comes in on the third day after childbirth. The boiled cow's milk and supplemental rice water worked very well. The infant mortality rate has been greatly reduced due to many innovative variables. The infant mortality rate is 93 infants die out of every thousand births (as of 2000).

Early one morning the bus pulled up outside the Maternity ward. A stretcher came out the back door carrying a woman in labor. They had traveled 50 miles and when she arrived the infant's head was visible. She had polio and when I attempted to examine, her, my students pulled her very contracted legs apart for the exam. Her legs were so stiff that they snapped back immediately around my waist. The infant had died and I began to cry in sympathy with her. She said "Don't cry Momma, there is another baby inside." She had been told by the village midwife that she was having twins. We could not hear the other fetal heartbeat. After the delivery of the dead infant, we examined her and waited – no signs of anything. It turned out she didn't have a twin but a tumor. It was a sad day.

Good Food, Good Friends

When I first arrived in Jinja, I went to the local catechumenate to hear the local dialect. It was conducted by the White Fathers and Brothers and local clergy. It was a good place to learn the local dialect and customs.

One day when we were all at break, several of the children spotted this mound in the ground and dug it up quickly. The children squealed in delight. It was the Queen Ant. They ran and gathered around the huge ant and proceeded to eat her. She was filled with millions of eggs which were high in protein and a delicacy (so they told me). I have eaten lion, Nile perch, fish of various sizes, warthog, tough chickens and beef, rabbits, kob, water buffalo, frogs and grasshoppers, but never the Queen Ant.

The good times were many and we made fast friends, which will be remembered all my life. Those were the days, my friend. In Jinja, near the hospital, was the Denbe Hotel, the local watering hole. They served mandazi (which is a donut-like sweet bread), matooke (steamed green bananas), meat and fish sauces. They served beer, Fanta, and Pepsi. In fact, Amin's mother's name was Fanta. She was always misnamed in the local press and called Pepsi.

One time I flew into Ethiopia to visit a hospital there to get ideas for change in our Ugandan Jinja Hospital. We were taken out to dinner by government officials to an Ethiopian restaurant for a real treat. They served meat and vegetables, deliciously cooked with special spices.

The meat, fish, etc. were laid out on Injira bread, a soft sour flat bread. The bread was in the form of a chapatti and filled the whole top of the basket table. We would tear off the bread and dip it in the sauces that were just laid on the bread using no utensils. No matter where you are in the world the company of good friends during an enjoyable time together enhances all foods. If you experience food, you truly share in their culture.

Shortage of Help

Ann was a local principal at one of the private schools. She was British and married a Ugandan and became a Ugandan citizen. At the time of this incident she had five children. She lived behind the hospital. We did not have a telephone in the nurses' hostel and the cell phone was a thing of the future. Ann appeared frantic at the door of the nurses' hostel with her flaccid one year old in her arms. He was not breathing.

I grabbed the infant from his mother's arms, spoke to the mother to drive to the maternity unit, and I ran to the unit myself all the while doing CPR and pumping the infant with my chest as I ran. I blew into his mouth after every five compressions.

When I arrived at the maternity unit, I continued into the Labor Room and placed the child on the slanted resuscitation board. We suctioned, took his vital signs and found 105 degree temperature. We immediately gave intramuscular Penicillin from Russia. The child responded and gradually started breathing on his own. Before we gave him the injection, we catheterized him to get a urine specimen. His fever was due to a urinary tract infection. The mother was very grateful, but I was reprimanded by the Pediatrician for giving the penicillin without a physician's written order.

There were no pediatricians available – they were all at the Crested Crane Hotel, and the attending physician was comfortable at home about 10 miles away. The child survived and eventually went on to college.

I do not want to give a negative impression of all the Ugandan physicians. I had many good experiences assisting and working with them. But thirty years ago with the political experiences that we all lived through and the availability of alcohol, often we could not get some of the doctors to come on duty and leave The Crested Crane Hotel. It put a lot of responsibility on the nursing staff.

One of the unforgettable doctors that I worked with in Jinja was a polio victim. I'll never forget the day we called him at the Doctor's Mess to come quickly to Labor and Delivery. It was the height of the rainy season and the hills to the Obstetric Ward were very muddy. Even with the assistance of his cane, he slipped and fell into the mud. When he finally arrived, he was covered with mud, and the baby, who had been lying in the transverse position in the mother's uterus, had been rotated and delivered by the staff midwives. He looked so dreadful and was very apologetic. Teamwork was always our goal.

Medical Safari

Medical safaris were always a lot of work, as well as a social event to meet the new expatriate doctors from China and various other countries worldwide. The medications given were from Russia and China. At that time, the Chinese workers were building the roads and training the Ugandan army.

When we went on safari in the Fort Portal area, I worked as a recording clerk, as I was not a nurse yet. This gave me an opportunity to visit the local homes and share their food, as well as get to know the translators. Hundreds of families would come to the Land Rover for physician exams and immunizations for their children.

After I trained as a nurse and midwife in England, I returned to experience a medical safari from the other end of the spectrum. We worked from sun up to sun down examining and training families from hundreds of miles around Jinja. We found that instead of two to three children, mothers would have six to seven children to continue the family. Many would lose four to five children to measles and sub-tropical diseases.

Medical Anomaly

At Jinja Hospital, one infant was born with such an anomaly that none of the staff would handle or take care of this baby girl. I had to get up in the middle of the night, go to the maternity, bathe and feed her. Her name was Sarah. We had to send one of the second year interns to Mulago Hospital and Makerere University in Kampala to do research, as to what was her diagnosis.

The signs were no eyelids and the skin would break open in dry cracks and she would bleed. None of the staff would touch her, as they thought they would catch whatever she had. When the intern returned from doing his research he found out what we were dealing with. The diagnosis was Congenital Icthiosis (icth - is Greek for fish). Skin scales and lack of eyelids were very conclusive.

Our plan of care started with isolation of the infant to stop the villagers lining up to view the patient and give the parents privacy and respect for their family care. Next we had to educate the staff that this disease was not contagious.

Then the family problems began. The father accused the mother as being the cause of the disease. He proceeded to start divorce proceedings immediately. When the standard of care was formalized, we called the local priest and social worker to work with the family for counseling.

Cleanliness and I.V. antibiotic therapy continued for three days. The priest was called and baptism was given to Sarah. She died on the third day. Everyone agreed that it was a very sad lesson for us all in the reverence we should all have for all forms of life.

Fear of the Night

I remember well the Ugandan fear of the night. We never went out after dark. The main Jinja Hospital was a mile from the donated dental clinic that we had turned into a children and isolation ward. If there was a seriously ill child that came to the children's ward during the night, the child really had to be very seriously ill for the parents to travel in the dark.

The charge nurse would call the Doctors Mess; describe the signs and symptoms to the doctor and take verbal orders. The child would be seen by the doctor first thing in the morning.

There were, however, exceptions to this practice. After learning the language and culture of Uganda, I went on duty 24/7 (on-call). There was a State Research man (Intelligence) who was assigned to watch me day and night as they were not sure yet what my role here was. I knew who he was and what he was doing. He did not make a game of it. When I was in Labor and Delivery, he was right outside the door. The staff inquired as to whether his presence bothered me at all. I told them, "What a waste of time for that individual. I was simply there for the mothers and children."

I would often get up in the middle of the night to go to Labor and Delivery if the midwife was having trouble. One night at 2a.m., there he was following me again. I asked him to walk with me instead of behind me for safety. Finally, one night he stated that he had spoken to his supervisor and told him of the good work that I was doing. He also stated that he had become exhausted doing the 24 hour duty. Once it was determined that I was not a threat, he left to the cheering of the staff. He departed without my knowing his name.

A young intern told me from his hospital bed that he had gone on his bike to see his girlfriend after dark. She refused to let him in as she was entertaining another friend. As he attempted to leave the compound he heard a war cry from the locals, as they came after him with their pangas (large knives). They thought he was a thief attempting to steal their bicycles. No questions asked, they cut off his ear and beat him to unconsciousness. Later that morning I was told that a doctor had been admitted to the men's surgical ward. I went to visit and could not find him. He called out to me from the main ward and was unrecognizable.

The Local Market

One of the simple pleasures of living in Uganda was the local market. Where in the world would I ever see such color? I had a few coins in my pocket and a few friends on a Saturday afternoon. We entered the market and surveyed the scene. There was row after row of colorful African prints laid out on the reddish-orange soil. The produce was everything from pineapples to vegetables and wonderful colored curries, to water pots, tire-soled shoes and jewelry. We meandered up and down the aisles choosing what little we could afford. The market was always a place for conversation and meeting former patients who were all well now, as well as patients who were still in their hospital gowns who were shopping for their hospital supper. Hospital food was provided but most patients supplemented from extras from the market. I never said anything to them but was just grateful that it was the right food group that they were buying.

When I returned to the United States there was a package waiting for me. It was wrapped in newspaper (The Voice of Uganda) and was tied with sewing thread. As I opened it carefully, I wondered how many miles it had traveled and when it had been posted. Inside the package there were ten small packs of different colored curries. My students had thought I would be lost without the curry flavor in my stew.

Mrs. Meredith

When I was in Fort Portal for a while, I felt comfortable navigating the dirt roads by myself. One such walk was down the road to Mrs. Meredith's house for Sunday tea. Mrs. Meredith had been in Uganda for fifty years and when I knew her she was 85 years old. She had been married to her husband on a boat riding up the Nile River. She had been married to him for over 40 years.

I always enjoyed entering her house for the Sunday afternoon tea. Outside it looked like a large African shamba, mud walls and a grass roof; but when you entered you thought you were in southern England. Everything was complete from the rugs to the English furniture. She served us tea and scones with guava jelly. She had grown the tea on her own plantation, which she tended for fifty years. When I had first met her, she had given the daily harvesting duties to the Ugandans.

She even grew the guava and made her own jelly. Every time I ate the scones and guava jelly, exactly one hour later I had to excuse myself and go to the powder room. The scones remained inside; but I was separated from the guava jelly. Can you imagine how selective our bodies are?

Common Sense

I used to teach common sense and assertiveness to my Post-Graduate Pediatric students. This came into play when the stool specimens were collected early every morning like clockwork. Patients were charged for their lab tests so we tried as best we could to keep the bills down. One of these students asked if it was reasonable to take the tapeworm to the lab in the cup and lid when it was so vigorous that it used to tip the lid off. We met with the doctors and took a vote. If the parasite was visible, viable and identifiable it did not have to go the lab but could be signed off by the doctors and the nurses. It all involved teamwork.

Child Pilot

On one of my trips to Arua, northern Uganda, we had toured the hospital and had meeting after meeting. I was now ready to go home to Jinja and was the only passenger on the plane. As we took off on the grass runway, we hit some turbulence and the door of the pilot's cabin flew open. I took a good look into the cockpit. I could not believe my eyes. The "pilot" at the controls was a fourteen-year old child. As I looked further into the co-pilot's seat I saw a BOAC pilot a lot older. I was so relieved to see a more experienced pilot on board. I have flown all over the world and have always been impressed by the safety and skills of the flight crew and pilots.

Rough Return to the U.S.

In 1979 when I flew back to America after my recuperation in England, I longed to see my parents. I had received weekly air letters from them while in Uganda. Near the end of my time there, I noticed the shakiness of my father's handwriting. I knew this was the beginning of his Parkinson's disease. All of this information combined with the dangers cropping up in Uganda was the final impetus for me to go.

We flew from Heathrow Airport in London. It was a quiet, uneventful flight. As we flew over the airport of our final destination in New York City, the pilot could not get the landing gear down. I thought "What an end to a decade of flying." I had flown all over the world landing on tarmac, grass, sand and water. And here on the last journey, we had no landing gear. We heard a flurry of activity below the floor of the plane. We heard the pilot order the dumping of the fuel as we continued to circle the airport. We flew out to sea where the dumping of the fuel occurred. I can always remember the assertiveness and kindness of the stewardesses. They told us the truth and took us through the emergency landing procedures. We were going to land on foam and skid down the runway to a stop. They explained that we would be using the rubber ramps to disembark once we came to a full stop. But most important of all, they communicated with us in a calm, organized way.

I always remember this strategy when communicating with families whose loved ones had taken a turn for the worst.

A "Hail Mary Pass"

I have long been a fan of Notre Dame football. Football strategies never leave your subconscious mind. This went into play when I was presented in the Labor and Delivery room with a fourteen-year old, three foot tall, Pygmy woman – child. She had been brought to our hospital since the village midwife could not manage her behavior. When she arrived, I immediately saw why. We could not even get close enough to give her pain medication.

At that time we had no linens or mattresses. The patient brought them from home for delivery. The little girl was all over the room. When we asked her to slow down and lie on the bed, she bounced up and down on the bedsprings. I knew this was an impossible position for delivery.

So we compromised. We built a nest of our own pillows and blankets on the floor and I used the Swahili word for "squat". This position is the most utilized in the world. Most primitive women prepare a hole in the ground and line it with rabbit fur. They squat over the hole to deliver their infants. The infant comes out and then the placenta is delivered and covers the infant in warmth as the cord is separated. The cord is milked for extra blood from the placenta into the infant before the ceremony of cutting the cord.

90

This was her first infant and we had a lot of teaching to do. Immediately, as primitive as she was, I could see the bonding with infant begin.

After discharge, she faithfully brought the infant back for immunizations, checkups and weighing of the infant in a swing. This swing was attached to a scale hung on a tree (similar to scales that we have in the U. S. for weighing vegetables).

As the child continued to gain weight and was breastfed every three hours, her mother worked on the hills of the tea plantation. Her child did come into the clinic but was never admitted to the hospital with a serious disease.

That is called my "Hail Mary Pass".

A Friend Indeed

We tried to run hospitals with practically nothing. Sometimes the electricity would go out during surgeries and deliveries. Shortages of medical supplies, especially medications, were a daily occurrence. At one time Gentamycin was the only antibiotic in the whole country. It was a cause of many children going deaf, as a side effect.

But we all get by with a little help from our friends. I met Helen Wagabaza in August 1976 as I was begging for sugar for the children's porridge. I was introduced to Paul, her husband, later. Helen and Paul had been students at Wisconsin University at Steven's Point where they married, had two children and moved to Uganda. Helen was a Jehovah's Witness and a U.S. citizen and Paul was Catholic and Ugandan. For Helen, when they returned to Uganda, it had been sight unseen. Helen worked at the local sugar refinery business and Paul taught Art at the local secondary school.

Every time we talk on the phone, Helen reminds me not to forget the story of her daughter Rachael's burn. I endeared myself to them when Rachael, a toddler, pulled a teacup with scalding tea and milk onto her chest. Her mother was very distressed and we gave treatment quickly. There was no scarring to the great relief of Helen. We remained friends and when I escaped in January 1979, this family followed me to Kenya by way of train and eventually to the United States of America. Of my 3,500 deliveries I delivered two of Helen's children. Daniel was born in August 1977 and David was born November 1978. Sarah, the eighth child, was born in the United States. My godchildren, Matia, Timmy, Charles, Lisa, Rachael, Daniel, David and Sarah have all heard stories from their parents about the suffering, but also about the joyful times they had all endured in their beloved country.

The Escape

How did I know when to go? After years of learning how to listen and watch carefully, I knew when everything came together. I truly got by with a little help from my real friends.

The rumors soon turned true and people said to me it would not be safe for me to wear my white nurses' uniform and cap any longer, as I was a conspicuous target. The dances at the local barracks with my friend Julianna, the head of the Girl Guides, soon came to an end. My movements were also limited. Hospital Administrators tried to keep me on the main compound; but I had to transport the sterilized bottles of I.V. fluids on my bike a mile to the children's hospital when the Land Rover was on safari. The I.V. fluids were mixed in the pharmacy in glass bottles, sterilized by autoclave in the Central Supply, and transported by Land Rover or me by bike to the isolation children's ward where most of the children were seriously ill. I started giving away my personal possessions slowly and very quietly. The recipients were sworn to secrecy. My dishes and cookware went to one of the doctors and his fiancé. My little hot plate and oven, good for cooking rabbit, went to Toppy, my dear friend. She never lied to me; I trusted her implicitly. The small refrigerator went to the children's ward to store immunizations. My clothing was given to my students, the post-graduate pediatric students. My bike went to Luka, a laundry worker, who had assembled my bike when I first arrived.

The money had gradually been withdrawn from the local Barclay's Bank and distributed according to the need I saw. My bank had sent one third of my salary to London, thirty pounds monthly. The other two thirds basically went for school fees for Stella Maris, an orphaned child raised at Jinja Hospital.

Another problem that bothered me was the missing salaries of my students from their exchange work done in Libya. Now there were no diplomatic relations between Uganda and Libya and the money remained in Libya. I had copied the bank account numbers of the students that were due this money for future reference.

I decided to stop over in Libya on my way home to see if I could get some answers from Mumammar Al-Qaddafi who had traded "slave labor" in the form of my students for a plane full of antibiotic fluids destined for Uganda.

The students came to me the previous year with their letters of appointment for up-grading in Libya. "Momma Mary," they shouted, "we are going to Libya for up-grading!" I painfully drew a darker picture for them and it turned out that I was right. They were used by the Libyan government to deliver the babies of the Muslim women. The Ugandans were not allowed to drink any alcohol in a Muslim country. They used to ferment their bananas in their closets for their banana beer. When I finally arrived in Libya, I went from department to department and finally got their money transferred to Uganda.

Julianna Bezuidenhout (her mother was African and her father was Dutch) and a White Brother from the United States were my basic escape crew. It took us three weeks to plan as Uganda was gradually disintegrating into war. The Land Rover pulled up to the nurses' hostel at 6am in the bright sunlight. We all hugged and I was gone.

Our road trip to the Ugandan-Kenya border was uneventful with one stop to buy a sheepskin hat. Could you imagine that – sheepskin hats were sold at a roadside stall. It served me well when I stayed for three months recovering in England.

When we arrived at the border, we were all fearful of what awaited us. It could go either way. As we drove up, there was no one there. We went through and found out later that there had been an uprising in Kampala and the border guards had left early in the morning to check about their families in Kampala. I had been very concerned about how I would cross the border since I had broken my contract, not paid my taxes, and was in fear for my life.

My open airline ticket to London was in my shoe, along with some notes with information for later use. My friend Helen in Jinja had purchased the ticket for me in Kenya when she had gone for medical treatment. My six hundred dollars had served me well. I was free. When we arrived at Julianna's sister's flat in Kenya, I slept for three solid days. When I finally awoke, we went to the airport and scheduled my airline ticket for one week later.

On the road between the Uganda border and Nairobi, we stopped to eat lunch and heard a loud noise coming over the hill. It was the beginning of a line of tanks coming from Kenya to invade the border of Uganda.

There were huge turrets and the driver and company were all drunk. All I could think about was getting out of there fast before someone hit the red button and finished us all off.

As I listened to the television in Nairobi when I was resting, we had uncensored news that I had not heard in years. I never knew what danger we were all in. The black and white pictures in the local newspapers of the dead bodies were so very stark in the familiar environments known to us. We even recognized some of the bodies.

Amin was running and hiding from Entebbe to Kampala to Jinja. Every so often a quote of his would appear in The Voice of Uganda in an attempt to cover for his lack of control. One of his absurd sayings comes to my mind, "If you have an itch on your behind, it will follow you wherever you go."

On my trip to Kenya, I carried my farewell gift from my students. It was a water pot made from the mud of the Nile River. My students made a donut cushion out of banana fiber and plaited banana fibers for the handle. This pot traveled with me 8,000 miles and never broke because it was well cushioned. I carried it wherever I went. The students purchased the water pot at the local market and were given strict instructions how to care for it.

They gave me all the instructions as I was leaving but I really did not pay much attention, as I was very anxious to leave. I guess it looked strange to all of the passengers on the plane as I tried to fit it in the overhead compartment. It traveled with me through Uganda, Kenya, England and finally to the United States. My parents laughed when I finally put water and flowers into it and found out that it leaked. Only then did I remember the instructions, "Be patient, the water pot will leak at first until the mud seals itself off." How true that was!

Now, when I hear all the instructions for embarking on a plane I can only think of the age of innocence in flying thirty years ago. One time when I was returning to Uganda after a furlough of three months, I had received a supply of disposable scissors, forceps, etc. that we could sterilize for reuse. I packed these "disposables" and filled five suitcases. I had no idea how I was ever going to pay for this overweight.

I just knew that I had to wear my white nurses' uniform and white cap and all of my nursing medals. When I arrived at the airline check-in desk, they weighed everything, as I was telling the airline personnel about my work and the terrible need in Uganda. Something told me to flash my medals I flashed and they let me go for nothing – just a lot of good will. Imagine that happening in today's world!

As Julianna, Paul (the White Brother), and I drove to the Kenya border, I could not help remembering all of the great times we had together. I especially remember in my prayers the Ugandan woman who died on the delivery table from a massive heart attack and severe anemia. We performed CPR for a long time to no avail. Her infant's heartbeat remained strong as the midwives performed a C-Section--no doctors available, of course-- and delivered a beautiful, healthy baby boy. Her relatives thought sadly of the mother's life and death; but rejoiced in her newborn son – life truly coming after death.

On Uganda's Terms

The Lessons

In America, all of our senses are truly the best entertained, and the least fulfilled is our dignity and safe health practices.

In April 1980, a Philadelphia Inquirer's newspaper article by Ray Moseby was entitled "A Year After Amin, Uganda's Struggle to Mend Itself." And so it continues to mend until this very minute.

The article goes on to state what was happening in a small town in southern Uganda by the name of Masaka. It stated that the white cement floors on the Masaka city hall lay shattered and compressed together like a huge three-layer cake, just as they were after a Tanzanian artillery barrage flattened the building in February of 1979. We used to travel there by Land Rover on safari and it was always a hub of activity. The Tropic Inn Hotel just like many other hotels all over Uganda was a roofless, burnt out shell.

At the army barracks west of town, once the headquarters of Dictator Idi Amin's elite suicide squad division, a comical looking stone lion looks out over the broken remains of a dozen army vehicles and the ruined walls of the barracks. So it is over all of Masaka.

A city of almost 200,000 a year ago is now a village of just 10,000 people whose stark ruins remind us of European cities after World War II.

Approximately 95% of the buildings are damaged or destroyed. Masaka, capital of Uganda's once rich coffee growing region, seems to be a city frozen in time. A year after the overthrow by Amin nothing has been done about rebuilding Masaka. It's a good question when anything will be.

Devastated by eight years of Amin's tyranny and by the war that brought about his downfall, the country that Winston Churchill called "The Pearl of Africa's Crown" remains virtually paralyzed with most of the money going to the central government and people utilizing subsistence farming.

The potential is tremendous. Uganda has some of the richest soil in the world; its mineral wealth still to be determined. Nineteenth century explorers found the people to be among the most intelligent and advanced in Africa, and that judgment holds firm even today.

The factories that were looted during the war against Amin are just coming back to work in this century. Hundreds of shops in Kampala, the capital, stand deserted, their windows smashed by looters in 1979 and not yet replaced as of 1980 (Kampala is completely refurbished as of 2007).

Cash crops that once earned millions of dollars, such as sugar, cotton and tobacco, are hardly grown any more. Meager foreign exchange reserves are being spent to import them.

Coffee, almost alone, carries the economy, accounting for 97% of export earnings. But production is down by a third and millions of dollars worth of coffee is being smuggled abroad and sold on the black market.

Many of the coffee growers are having a very hard time surviving. They have no insecticides so the coffee dies. They have no hoes and tractors and transportation is a serious problem.

During the 1980's schools, highways, hospitals, trucks and buses are all in deplorable condition. Kampala, just 20 miles from Lake Victoria, is without water supplies much of the time because of a breakdown in pumping equipment.

Eighty percent of the Ugandan labor force is unemployed (1980). Only the countries fertile soil prevents widespread starvation. Those without work simply go back to their villages and get by on subsistence farming.

A large part of Uganda's problem is money. But another part is a government that is torn by factional squabbling and corruption and has proved unable to come to grips with the country's problems.

A disillusioned official who returned from exile after Amin's overthrow said, "There is corruption at the top of the government, and there is a widespread feeling that the government is not working for the people. We need to have a moral rehabilitation before we can have a structural rehabilitation."

With goods in short supply, Uganda's money is worth only one-tenth of its official value. Sometimes prices are up as much as one hundred percent. Incomes are fixed at low levels, corruption has become a way of life for thousands of Ugandans. It takes such forms as smuggling, pilfering, illegal currency dealing and bribe taking.

Symptomatic of the government's approach to problems was a recent decision allocating ten million dollars to Roman Catholics to make pilgrimages to Rome and Lourdes. Emmanuel Cardinal Nsubuga, Archbishop of Kampala, is reported to have demanded the funds to redress an inequity that occurred under Amin, a Muslim. At that time, Catholics were not allowed to go on pilgrimages but Muslims were given funds to go to Mecca. In 1978 the head nurse from the maternity went to Mecca with a large group of Muslims. She left me in charge of the premature baby unit and the maternity ward. I had to hire an indigenous Ugandan who really knew the staff and customs to take care of staffing problems, as the staff would approach me and want time off for the death of their mother (who had died three times previously). And so the lies continued.

The internal security situation, although far from ideal, has improved. Towards the end of 1979, shootings in Kampala became less frequent. In 1980 all of the Tanzanians were gone, their places taken by a newly trained Ugandan army that initially totaled 10,000 men.

Perhaps the most important sign of progress is that the government decided to hold national elections in December 1980. These elections were Uganda's first in 18 years, and were regarded by diplomats as a vital step in ending political bickering and achieving political stability. When the displaced Ugandans returned to their burnt out villages and homes, many commented that not even a bird sang when they returned to rebuild.

As the Tanzanians withdrew, another terror was invading Uganda in the form of a disease that is worldwide. AIDS had not been officially diagnosed until 1984 although the symptoms first appeared in 1980, one year after my escape. In Robert Caputo's article in National Geographic Magazine, "Land Beyond Sorrow", I first read about "Slim". That's what the Ugandans called AIDS. They used this word because of the skeletal appearance of the victims in the last stage of the disease.

AIDS had reached epidemic proportions in Uganda in which perhaps 800,000 people had been slaughtered in twenty years of intermittent civil war. The breakdown of communications and healthcare systems make it impossible to compile reliable numbers, but informed sources stated that one in every five sexually active adults in Kampala, the capital, are infected (between 18 to 40 years of age). Most AIDS patients are cared for by their families. The spread is mainly through heterosexual intercourse and affects men and women equally. Rumors say that about 40% of all Ugandans are positive for AIDS.

Fighting an epidemic of ignorance along with the disease, Ugandans and WHO officials train lab technicians from remote districts to help prevent AIDS. Workers with the Institute of Public Health, Makerere University, collect data for regional surveys, interview Ugandans about their sexual practices, and take blood for testing. They also distribute educational leaflets and counsel Ugandans to "Love Carefully".

According to the "Facts About Uganda" released by the Ugandan Embassy, in 1985 the population was 15,500,000 with a literacy rate of 52% and life expectancy of 50 years.

Small stands along the dirt roads, originally built to display tomatoes, bananas, and other produce exhibited human skulls gathered from the killing fields.

A National Committee for the Prevention of AIDS is in place, as is a program coordinated by WHO, to which donor nations have pledged millions for education, medical equipment and supplies. Public meetings are held to discuss AIDS, and a curriculum incorporating AIDS education has been prepared for the schools. Warning leaflets have been printed in ten languages. Slogans of the campaign are "Love Carefully" and "Zero Grazing" (an agricultural metaphor).

The second largest category, about 10%, is the transmission of AIDS from mother to infant. There are some transmissions through blood transfusions and unsterilized needles but Ugandans access to healthcare has been so disrupted that these play a marginal role.

AIDS was first noted in Uganda in early 1980 by people in a small fishing and smuggling village along Lake Victoria. Smuggling was a major economic activity, and these mud-hut villages throbbed with commerce. Boats traveled between Uganda, Tanzania and Kenya, and lorries traveled along the roads between Uganda, the Democratic Republic of the Congo, and Rwanda. Bars and hotels sprang up, local breweries went into production – and prostitutes by the hundreds descended on the lake giving service to the free-spending, hard-drinking traders.

According to the theory, the traders returned to their homes carrying the organism with them, as did the truck drivers from as far away as Mombassa, on the Indian Ocean. These men infected their wives, lovers, or other prostitutes who passed the organism on to their partners. The lines of AIDS concentration in central and eastern Africa followed very closely those of commerce.

AIDS is not limited to the high-risk group of prostitutes and truck drivers. It has been reported in every district of Uganda, and it strikes farmers and townspeople alike.

The first case was officially diagnosed in 1984 in an area west of Lake Victoria – where most people eke out meager livings on small farms scattered across the countryside.

When the villagers first noticed the disease, they thought it was witchcraft. They believed the Tanzanians were cursing people who had cheated them. I remember at Jinja Hospital when I worked as a nurse, a man died of fright (heart attack) when he took his shirt from the wash line and found a small postage stamp piece had been cut out of the collar. Apparently he thought that one of his enemies had taken the piece of cloth to the witch doctor for a curse.

This society can be summed up in their reluctance to change behavior. One man stated that a man has a wife and a woman has a husband, but they also have many, many good friends.

Most of the people in the farming areas spend all of the daylight hours digging in their fields, and doing the chores – fetching water and firewood, and cooking – that enables them to survive. It is a hard existence with few rewards.

News came from the oasis of agriculture near the Rwenzori Mountains in Fort Portal. Workers at the Kahuna Tea Estate had reclaimed fields overgrown during the years of war reopened by a British firm in partnership with Uganda. Kahuna is one of the many foreign-owned plantations confiscated by Idi Amin in 1972.

Tea, coffee and cotton all grow well in Uganda. In Fort Portal, we fenced in an area with wooden stakes. They sprouted into a fence of trees. That is how fertile the soil is. Economists say that unlike famine-stricken African countries, Uganda has resources to rebuild its economy given a few years of peace.

Most cars are in poor condition, the roads horrible, and the people drive as though someone is after them.

The refugees tried to get on the road to a normal life by crossing the border between Sudan and Uganda. They had fled for their lives during Obote's second try at the presidency. Their aim was to get back to their homes in the northern Nile province.

The Ugandan High Commission for Refugees operates tribal camps and reception centers, where returning refugees are given food, blankets, and farm tools to help them rebuild their lives. More than one million Ugandans were displaced between 1980 and 1985.

Death on wheels was a common sight where Ugandans shrouded a dead body in bark cloth and placed it across the handlebars of their bicycles to move it to its final resting place in fields outside the town.

Uganda struggles to find signs of hope in lands where a vision of hell has become commonplace.

In 1986, the Ugandan population was estimated to be 15.1 million. In 2000 another estimate was 23,317,560. In 2005, the UN estimated 27.6 million people. The life expectancy is 46 years for men and 47 years for women based on UN statistics.

Tourism in Uganda has been very slow to return due to security issues. In Uganda's "Visit Uganda" website on tourism they state, "From the moment you land at

Entebbe's modern and efficient international airport, with its breathtaking equatorial location on the forested shore of an island-strewn Lake Victoria, it is clear that Uganda is no ordinary safari destination. Dominated by an expansive golf course leading down to the lakeshore, and a century old botanical garden alive with the chatter of acrobatic monkeys and colorful tropical birds, Entebbe itself is the least obviously urban of all comparably sized African towns. Then, just 40 kilometers distance, sprawled across seven hills, there is the capital Kampala. The bright modern feel of this bustling, cosmopolitan city reflects the ongoing economic growth and political stability that has characterized Uganda since 1986, and is complemented by the sloping spaciousness and runaway greenery of its garden setting.

Ecologically, Uganda is where the East African savannah meets the West African jungle. Where else but in this impossibly lush country can one observe lions prowling the open plains in the morning and track chimpanzees through the rain forest undergrowth the same afternoon, then the next day navigate tropical channels teeming with hippo and crocs before setting off into the misty mountains to stare deep into the eyes of a mountain gorilla? Certainly, Uganda is the only safari destination whose range of forest primates is as impressive as its selection of plains antelope. And this verdant biodiversity is further attested to by Uganda's status as by far the smallest of the four African countries whose bird checklist tops the thousand mark!

Yet there is more to the country than wildlife – far more! There is the mighty Nile, punctuated by the spectacular Murchison Falls and the setting for some of the world's most thrilling commercial whitewater rafting.

There are the snow-capped peaks of the Rwenzori, which provide a tantalizing challenge to dedicated mountaineers, as well as the Birunga Volcanoes and Mount Elgon, both of which offer highly rewarding hiking opportunities through scintillating highland scenery. More sedately, the myriad island of Lake Victoria and Bunyonyi are idyllic venues as are the myriad forest-fringed crater lakes that stud the rift valley floor and escarpment around Fort Portal. Whether you are a first time safari-goer or a seasoned African traveler, Uganda – with its unique blend of savannah and forest creatures, its rare wealth of African habitats – is simply dazzling.

Uganda's reputation as 'Africa's Friendliest Country' stems partly from the tradition of hospitality common to its culturally diverse population, and partly from the remarkably low level of crime and hassle directed at tourists. But this amicable quality extends beyond the easygoing people. Uganda's eco-friendliness is attested to by the creation of six new national parks under the present administration, as well as a recent mushrooming of community-based eco-tourism projects at the grassroots level, while the mood of social enlightenment is characterized by the progressive and much lauded policies towards curbing the spread of HIV/AIDS and promoting women's rights. The climate, too, is highly agreeable, reflecting the combination of equatorial location and medium to high altitudes, while amenities such as hotels and game lodges now rank with the very best Africa has to offer."

According to the BBC news "Country Profile: Uganda" main exports are coffee, fish and fish products, tea, tobacco, cotton, corn, beans, and sesame.

Agriculture is the main industrial activity: coffee is the main export crop. Uganda is the world's second largest producer of coffee. Uganda has posted a gross domestic product growth rate above 5% for ten years in a row. The GDP was estimated at 24.2 billion dollars in 1999. The 1999 estimated GDP per capita was $1,060.

The fertility rate is seven children per woman. The literacy rate is 62% of people age 15 and above. School is in session almost all year with the exception to 2-3 weeks in May or August, part of December and all of January. School fees are a burden on everyone; but there are private organizations that help with the school fees. University is paid for by the government.

BBC News continues. Private radio and television stations have mushroomed since the government loosened its controls on the media in 1993. But, the state sometimes criticizes the conduct of some of the hundred or so private radio and television stations. Some have been accused of raising ethnic tensions and of being negative in their reporting. The authorities suspended broadcast of a popular service KFM for a time in August of 2005 after it broadcast a debate about the health of a Sudanese former rebel leader. Public UBC radio came to be heard across the country in English and vernacular languages. BBC World Services is widely available on FM Radio; France International broadcasts on FM in Kampala.

Although the print media is led by the state-owned New Vision newspaper, it enjoys considerable independence and often publishes articles which criticize the government.

"New Vision" reports, politically, the Republic of Uganda had its multi-party politics reinstated in 2005.

Regarding security, the government and the Lord's Resistance Army (LRA – cult-like) rebels have signed a truce aimed at ending a nineteen year conflict.

Regarding the economy, Uganda is vulnerable to changes in the world price of coffee, its main export product.

Internationally, Uganda has been actively involved in the Democratic Republic of the Congo conflict. LRA leaders are wanted by the International Criminal Court for war crimes.

Since becoming president in 1986, Yoweri Museveni has introduced democratic reform and has been credited with substantially improving human rights, notably by reducing abuses between the army and the police.

According to the Uganda Website, the Parliament of Uganda derives its mandates and functions from the 1995 Constitution, the Laws of Uganda and its own Rules of Procedure. The Constitution contains articles which provide for the establishment, composition and functions of the Parliament of Uganda and empowers Parliament "to make laws on any matter for peace, order, development and good governance of Uganda", and "to protect the Constitution and promote democratic governance in Uganda". The term of Parliament is five years from the date of its original first sitting after a general election. The current Parliament (8th Parliament) started in May 2006 and ends in May 2011.

The emphasis of the Ministry of Health lies in the concept of Public-Private Partnership is health increasing Private Health Sector participants in all aspects of the national health program.

The Public-Private Partnership in the Health Project was initiated in 1997 by the Ministry of Health. The proposal was forwarded through the Ministry of Economic Planning and Development to the Government of Italy. The implementation of the project commenced in July 2000 and is jointly funded by the Government of Uganda and the Government of Italy.

The Government aims to provide an enabling environment for the effective coordination of efforts among all partners, increase efficiency in resource allocation, achieve equity in the distribution of available resource for health-effective access by all Ugandans for essential healthcare.

In a world filled with disease, terrorism, dictatorships, drugs, prostitution, corruption and corporate vice, we have to be creative, knowledgeable, safe and not sorry.

I'll always remember the industry of the marching ants – the Queen Ant, her workers, her soldiers and her guardians. When we went on safaris, we would stop driving for a rest and walk into the surrounding areas to investigate. I wanted my picture taken sitting on a huge ant hill (three feet high). I no sooner sat on the top, when I was covered with the hills defense team of working ants. The itch went on for weeks.

I couldn't help remembering centuries ago when the pinchers on the soldier ants were used in surgically clamping the wound shut. Then the "surgeons" would pinch off the body of the ant and the pinchers would remain until the wound healed. We've come a long way! I learned my lesson well – never to interrupt the line of the marching ants.

This is well illustrated at Jinja Hospital when the mothers would wash out the children's clothing and lay it on the grass in front of the Nutrition Teaching Garden (Mwanamugimu – "you have fallen into good things"). At the height of the heat at noon, the clothes would be spotted moving across the lawn. The marching ants, again – you never disturb them – you just waited patiently until they got tired. Then you grabbed your clothes and ran.

On my way home I stopped off to recuperate in London and went by train to southern England to Hastings. I received the hospitality of Peggy Daly (retired) who was the Head of Nursing Education in Uganda under the British protectorate. I retrieved some of my weight loss and recovered my body and spirits while I stayed with Peggy Daly. She only knew the good times and we had many hours of reminiscence.

When I returned home, I stayed with my parents, who could not get over how much weight I had lost. My hands, from which I earned my living, looked like eighty year old hands. I used to eat the potato skins left over on my parents dinner plates as I could not stand to see any waste. To this day, I feed the birds the left over pizza crust.

I can't say I had a death wish when I left Uganda. However, after I reached home the amount of mail received from my students and other friends, requesting money, scholarships and hospitality, etc. was prohibitive. The "peculiar" mail and hang-up phone calls still fill me with terror. I had been so fearful over the years about the State Research Bureau, that terrors at any "odd event" registered that I might have been followed out of Uganda.

During the years that followed, I sent a message back to Uganda through my Ugandan friends' relatives that I had died. This seems to have been accepted.

Well, I am back and feel that thirty years is long enough to keep silent about the Ugandan people. I always felt protected by the ordinary people; perhaps I brought them a ray of hope.

The African world and the Western world are many worlds apart. But, we share our humanity in common.

Children are our treasures. In my various gatherings in the U.S., I am often asked how many children I have. I tell them 3,500 which accounts for all of my deliveries in England and Africa.

In conclusion, I think about the beginning words of the Preamble of our U.S. Constitution, "We, the people.....". What is our responsibility as citizens of a technologically advanced nation where information abounds?

On Uganda's Terms

References

1. BBC News: http://news.bbc.co.uk/90/pr/fr/-/1/n:/world/africa/country-profiles/1069166.stm; Published 2007/01/19.

2. Caputo, Robert, "Uganda – Land Beyond Sorrow", National Geographic Magazine, Vol. 173 No. 4, April 1988; pp. 468-491.

3. Daily Nation (Kenya), No. 5715, Wednesday, April 18, 1979.

4. "Facts About Uganda"; 3/26/02 Website http://www.ugandaembassy.org/ugandafacts.htm pp.1-3.

5. Foden, G., "The Last King of Scotland", 1998. Vintage International, A Division of Random House Inc., NY, NY.

6. Kakitahi, J., Dr., Lecturer, Makerere Institute of Public Health, "Food and Nutrition", Ministry of Health News Bulletin, Vol. No. 2, December, 1977, Ministry of Health, P.O. Box 8, Entebbe, Uganda, pp.10-11.

7. Kasumba, S.S., Dr., Administration/Public Health, "Handling and Administration of Measles Vaccine", Ministry of Health News Bulletin, Vol.1, No. 2, pp.13-14.

8. Maimonides, Rabbi Moses, 1963, "The Guide of the Perplexed", (Talmud), University of Chicago Press, Chicago, Illinois.

9. Miller, Barbara D., "Cultural Anthropology", 2nd Edition, 2002, Allyn & Bacon – A Pearson Education Company, Boston, MA, pp.12-26.

10. Ministry of Health Online, The Repulic of Uganda, "Public-Private Partnership in Health (PPPH): Increasing Private Health Sector Participaion in all Aspects of the National Health Programme, HTTP://www.health.go.reg/part-health.htm, Partnership in Health. Pp. 1-5.

11. Moseley, Ray (1980), "A Year After Amin, Uganda Struggles to Mend Itself", Vol. 300 No. 96, Chicago Tribune Service to The Philadelphia Inquirer Newspaper, April 6, 1980.

12. Musisi, Dr., Director of Medical Services of Uganda, "Cultural Social Beliefs and Behavior as a Factor in Prevention of Some Diseases in Mankind", Ministry of Health News Bulletin, Vol. 1, No. 2, December 1977. Ministry of Health, P.O. Box 8, Entebbe, Uganda, pp. 2-3.

13. Nanyonga, J. O., Health Education Office, "An Approach to Community Health Education", Ministry of Health News Bulletin, Vol. 1, No. 2, December 1977. Ministry of Health, P.O. Box 8, Entebbe, Uganda, pp. 8-9.

14. Nyabongo, Elizabeth (1989), "Elizabeth of Toro – An Autobiography, The Odyssey of an African Princess", Simon and Schuster Inc., NY, NY; London, England.

15. Okware, S., Dr., Ministry of Health Epidemiologist, "The Importance of the Venerial Disease Degree", Ministry of Health News Bulletin, Vol. 1, No. 2, December 1977. Ministry of Health, P.O. Box 8, Entebbe, Uganda, pp. 9-10.

16. Omara, A.B.M., Dr., "A Paper Presented by the Permanent Secretary Representing the Honorable Minister of Health (Idi Amin) at the Fifth Commonwealth Medical Conference in New Zealand on Food and Nutrition in Uganda", Ministry of Health News Bulletin, Vol. 1, No. 2, December 1977. Ministry of Health, P.O. Box 8, Entebbe, Uganda, pp. 4-8.

17. Parliament of Uganda Website, "About the Parliament (2006)", February 23, 2007, http://www.parliament.go.ug/indexphpoption=content andtask, p.1.

18. Time Magazine, "Tetanus Toxoid Vaccine: B. D. Uni-Ject Device", January 15, 2007, Vol. 164, No. 3, p.33, p.65.

19. Uganda Tourist Board, http:www.visituganda.com/elegant.html, Tourism Uganda – Uganda at a Glance, Uganda an Elegant Adventure.

20. Wellechinsky, D., (2007), "The World's Ten Worst Dictators", Philadelphia Inquirer Parade Magazine, Parade Publishing, NY, February 11, 2007.

Mary M. Hale, RN,C., MSN, SRN, SCM

EMPLOYMENT HISTORY

	Albert Einstein Medical Center, Philadelphia, PA
2003-2006	*Womens' and Childrens' Service Line (Maternity)*
1979-2003	*Pediatrics Unit*
	Jinja Hospital, Jinja, Uganda, East Africa
1976-1979	*Pediatrics and Neonatology Clinical Instructor – Day and Night Shifts*
	Wexham Park Hospital, Slough, Berks, Middlesex, England
1975-1976	*Pediatrics Charge Nurse*
	Hillingdon Hospital, Hillingdon, Uxbridge, Middlesex, England
1974-1975	*Obstetrics and Gynecology – Staff Midwife*
1972-1974	*Obstetrics and Gynecology – Student Midwife*

	Philadelphia General Hospital, Philadelphia, PA
	Detention Ward: Prisoners, Holmsburg Prison and Juvenile Detention Center
1972	*Staff Nurse*

EDUCATION

	LaSalle University, Philadelphia, PA
May, 1992	M.S.N. in Community Nursing
May, 1987	B.S.N. in Nursing

AWARDS

May, 1998	Research "Possible Quest" Contest – 1st Prize: "Normal Saline versus Heparin Saline Flushes for Pediatric Intermittent Intravenous Devices"
May, 1994	Research Recognition Award – Albert Einstein Medical Center, Philadelphia, PA
October, 1994	Pennsylvania Nurses' Association – Search for Excellence Award

ORGANIZATIONS

1990-1994	American Public Health Association

1986-1995	American Nurses' Association
1986-1995	Pennsylvania Nurses' Association

COMMITTEE/COUNCIL

MEMBERSHIPS

1990-1996	Quality Assurance Committee – Pediatrics Albert Einstein Medical Center, Philadelphia, PA
1990-1996	American Public Health Association – Community Health Planning and Policy Section
1988-1996	Research Council at Albert Einstein Medical Center, Philadelphia, PA

NURSING HONORS

SOCIETIES

1988-Present	Sigma Theta Tau – International Honor Society of Nursing
1986-Present	Alpha Epsilon – LaSalle University Honor Society
1986-Present	Kappa Delta – LaSalle University Nursing Honor Society

CERTIFICATION

1993-2006   Neonatal Advanced Life
             Support Certification

1993-2006   Pediatric Advanced Life
             Support Certification

1988-2006   Re-certification – Pediatric Nurse
             Child and Adolescent Nurse -
             #098258-07 American Nurses
             Credentialing Center

RESEARCH PROJECTS

April, 1998   **"Normal Saline Solution Versus
               Heparin Saline Flushes for Pediatric
               Intermittent Intravenous Devices:
               Safe and Economical for
               Pediatric Practice?"**
               First prize in "The Possible Quest"
               Research Contest – Albert Einstein
               Healthcare Network,Philadelphia, PA

February, 1996 **"The Comfort Basket – A Sign
               of the Times in Comfort Science"**
               A Pediatric Group Effort of
               Phenomological research entered
               into the "Possible Quest" contest –
               Albert Einstein Medical Center,
               Philadelphia, PA

1992-1994   **Thesis: "The Role of Locus of
               Control in Smoking Behavior"**

Sample: Community Focus – Mothers eligible for WIC Program.
Presented at: Albert Einstein Medical Center, Philadelphia, PA
Cooper Medical Center, New Jersey

PUBLICATIONS

2009   **On Uganda's Terms – 2nd Edition**
Hale, RNC, MSN, Mary M.
CCB Publishing

2008   **Beyond Nurses Notes**
Hale, RNC, MSN, Mary M.
CCB Publishing

2005   **Maternity Matters – Vol. 1-2**
Stories by AEMC Maternity Nurses in process of publication. To be incorporated into Dr. Sharon Hudacek's, Ph.D. book "Making a Difference: Stories from the Point of Care".

1998-2000   **Selected Tales from "The Comfort Basket" Published as Pediatric Chapter 5**
"Making a Difference: Stories from the Point of Care", Hudacek, Sharon PH.D, Center Nursing Press, A Division of Sigma Theta Tau International; Indianapolis, Indiana. pp. 60-69.

1997   **Dollops '97,** Vol. 4, No. 1, A Newsletter for Nurses, Provided by Astra USA,

Inc., "Comfort Basket and EMLA Cream Help Take Away Pediatric Pain". Authors: Mary M. Hale, RN,C., MSN and June Lowe, RN,C.

1996 **Albert Einstein Healthcare Network, "A Nurse is a Rare Combination"** – "Einstein Nurses…In Their Own Words" – "Tales from the Comfort Basket – The World of the Five Year Old" Author: Mary M. Hale, RN,C., MSN.

1995 **Nursing Times '95,** Albert Einstein Medical Center, "Crosstraining – A Journey of Rediscovery" Author: Mary M. Hale, RN,C., MSN.

1994 **Nursing Spectrum,** Vol. 3, No. 8, February 21, 1994: Nurse Entrepreneurs: "Clowning With a Difference" Authors: Tom Starner and Mary M. Hale, RN,C., MSN. An article about the beginnings of "Dear Lovely", the Delaware Valley's first Public Health – Teaching Clown for children and adolescents.

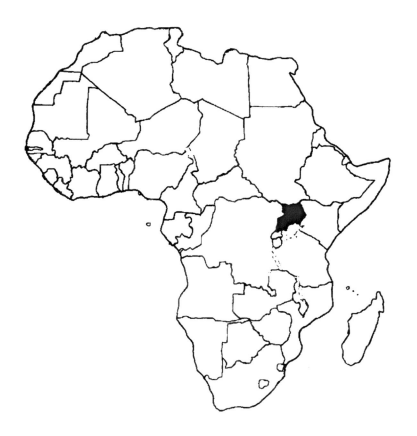

Thank you, Uganda!

Love & Humor have no borders.

– Mary –

CPSIA information can be obtained at www.ICGtesting.com
Printed in the USA
BVOW080459200313

315949BV00001B/40/P